We Band of Mothers: Autism, My Son and the Specific Carbohydrate Diet

We Band of Mothers: Autism, My Son and the Specific Carbohydrate Diet

By
Judith Chinitz, M.S.

With commentary by
Sidney M. Baker, M.D.

Autism Research Institute, San Diego

WE BAND OF MOTHERS: AUTISM, MY SON
AND THE SPECIFIC CARBOHYDRATE DIET

Copyright © 2007 by
Judith Chinitz, M.S., with commentary by Sidney M. Baker, M.D.

The views and opinions expressed by the contributors to this book are not
necessarily the views and opinions of the Autism Research Institute.

This book is not intended as medical advice. Its intention is solely informational and educational. Please consult a qualified medical or health professional if you wish to pursue
the ideas presented.

Neither the editors, contributors, nor the sponsoring organization, the Autism Research Institute, is engaged in rendering professional advice or services to the individual
reader. The ideas, procedures, and suggestions contained in this book are not intended as
a substitute for consulting with a qualified physician and obtaining medical supervision
regarding any activity, procedure, or suggestion that might affect your health. Neither the
editors, nor contributors, nor the sponsoring organization, shall be liable or responsible
for any loss, injury, or damage allegedly arising from any information or suggestion in this
book.

Published by the Autism Research Institute
4182 Adams Avenue
San Diego, CA 92116, U.S.A.
www.AutismResearchInstitute.com

ISBN 978-0-9740360-2-1

PRINTED IN THE UNITED STATES OF AMERICA

From this day to the ending of the world,
But we in it shall be remembered—
We few, we happy few, we band of brothers...

– From Shakespeare's *Henry V*

Table of Contents

For Alex, who gives me courage.

For Liam, who lights my way.

And for Elaine Gottschall and
Dr. Bernard Rimland—
my heroes.

Acknowledgments

My treat to myself upon finishing this book was to write this "thank-you" section. The opportunity to thank the important people in my life publicly has added impetus to get me to finish the writing as soon as possible.

I would never have survived this long with my sanity intact were it not for the incredible love and support of friends and family around me. The most wonderful people in the world are my parents, Dr. Wallace and Carol Chinitz, who have taught me that true love, in all its guises, is not a figment of the poetic imagination. Always there for me is my big brother, David (who's so great and nice and wonderful and intelligent), my sister-in-law, Lisa, and their children, Michael and Raina.

I want to thank Sid Baker, who has taught me that parents are the best source of clinical data, that wine is toxic fungal poison but who cares, and that I really do need to follow those who seek the truth and run from those who've found it…

And Dr. Marvin Boris, thank you. When I was a child you made going to the doctor something not to be dreaded. I would have guessed—even as a five year old (with a child's uncanny ability to recognize good)—that you'd still be there years later to help me and my family in our fight for health. You're everything a doctor should be.

Thank you to all of my old and wonderful friends, who are the wheat when the circumstances of my life separated them from the chaff—

thank you for not letting my grief drive you away.

And I have to thank the Dr. Moms, who embody the maternal ideal in their unwavering dedication, unconditional love, brilliance, drive, fortitude, and courage. To name but a few: there's Kate, who keeps me from putting my head in the oven by threatening to put her own in first. There's Jess, who lets me cry on her shoulder at any hour of the day and night, and whose warmth is a constant source of strength and comfort. There's Stacey, who constantly threatens to drag me to manicures and Starbucks—the cure for all ills. There are Candace and Heather, whose faces should be in the dictionary next to the word "courage." There's Martin (a Dr. Dad), whose SCD mayonnaise has earned him the illustrious title of Mayo Meister. There's Vanessa, who does a mean Inspector Clouseau imitation just to make me laugh. (What do you mean she really talks likes that?!) There's Jeannie, who unsuccessfully tries to hide her beauty and brilliance behind cowboy boots and Bud Lights, and who made me believe I really could write this book. To all of you Dr. Moms (and the Dr. Dad!): thank you for your friendship, for sharing your lives with me—and for casting someone who looks like Julia Roberts to play me in the movie.

Finally, I often remind myself at my darkest moments that there is more than one good thing I have gotten from Alex's illness. One of the greatest blessings was the honor of befriending truly great, truly towering human beings: Dr. Bernard Rimland and Elaine Gottschall. Their work has brought comfort and healing to countless thousands—not the least to me and my son. I find that the very thought of them renews my faith that in the end, maybe goodness really will prevail.

CHAPTER I

Alex's Story

Through me the way into the suffering city.
Through me the way to the eternal pain....
Abandon every hope, ye who enter here.

– On the gateway to hell, from Dante's *Inferno*

On March 22, 1996, my son, Alex, was diagnosed with autism. It was 19 days after his second birthday. I was with my mother at Mount Sinai Hospital in Manhattan when the developmental pediatrician shook his head and said, "Your story was excellently told. I have heard this story many times recently. Your son has a pervasive developmental disorder. He may continue to regress. We won't know where he is on this spectrum for a while yet."

I didn't really understand what he meant by a pervasive developmental disorder or spectrum. PDD wasn't yet a part of my vocabulary, even though I'd graduated with a Master's degree in special education only a few years earlier. It wasn't until I saw the neurologist, a few hours later, that I really understood what was going on.

My Alex. My love. My beautiful baby with his huge, blue eyes and thick, long, black lashes. Just saying his name even now causes a burst of heart-aching love to wash through me. For two years I watched him grow in beauty. And for one of those years I watched him leaving us, regressing into a world of his own, alone.

He was always a delicate baby, an exceptionally awful sleeper, a terrible eater. In fact, that first year of his life I'm not sure he ever slept for more than four or five hours in 24. He would not accept even baby foods, let alone solid foods, until he was nine months old. The slightest noise anywhere in our apartment would cause him to wake up, and he'd be awake for the next 18 or more hours.

His life didn't exactly start off on the right foot. At about 36 hours of age he developed a fever. Current medical protocol states that any baby under three months of age who develops a fever be hospitalized immediately and given intravenous antibiotics, just in case it's meningitis. After five days of hospitalization, with 24 hours a day of IV antibiotics, and even a spinal tap, Alex was in pretty poor shape. He refused to breastfeed anymore and ended up on formula after becoming dehydrated in the hospital. After that hospitalization, things were never right. As I said, he was a very delicate baby. But, again, in accordance with standard medical protocol, we proceeded with a normal vaccine schedule.

Things started to get worse and worse.

It wasn't until after we'd moved to England when he was twelve months old, however, that I started to get really worried. The first thing I noticed was that he'd stopped responding to his name when we went outside. When we first got to England, Alex would love to play "football" with me. I would put the ball between my legs, with him standing behind me, and I'd yell "7-14-21! HUT!" He would charge through my legs, grab the ball, and continue to run, laughing, until I tackled him. Then one day, he stopped playing. I would put the ball down to discover that he'd simply wandered off, and when I'd call to him, he wouldn't even turn around to look at me.

Next, he stopped responding to his name inside the house. No more games of peek-a-boo and hide-and-seek. I would try to get him to play but he'd simply sit there, a glazed, flat expression on his face, looking straight through me. Most of the time, he didn't seem to know there was another person there. He started to completely ignore us, simply sitting on the floor doing puzzles over and over for hours at a time.

I clearly remember sitting with him on the floor of our family room trying to get him to play with me, and his father coming home from work. "Alex!" he'd call, "Alex!" Our son wouldn't look up, wouldn't acknowledge that a person had entered the room, but would only proceed to put another piece in the puzzle he'd just done 20 times.

This is a story that has been told too many times by parents of kids in this epidemic of autism: losing our children, day by day, helplessly standing by while they vanish inside themselves. Twenty years ago, one in 10,000 children was diagnosed as autistic. When Alex was diagnosed in 1996 that number had risen to one in 500. Currently, that number is one in 150 children.

In Alex's case, his social withdrawal was accompanied by continually worsening health. With every day that passed, Alex became sicker and sicker.

And sicker.

Back to March 22, 1996, and our appointments at Mt. Sinai Hospital: I found out, subsequently, that neurologists are famous among doctors for being insensitive. At the time, however, I thought I was the lucky one to have been referred to this particular physician. Our appointment with him was the last in his day, on an afternoon during which he was due to leave for vacation. He made no attempt to disguise his impatience and irritation at having to spend those few minutes with us.

As I mentioned, we were living in England at the time, and I'd flown back to the U.S. with Alex the day before to make it to these appointments. He was exhausted, jet lagged, cranky, and we were in the hospital for hours, as there was a gap of about four hours between the appointments with the developmental pediatrician and the neurologist. By that time in his regression, Alex's best was never good, but when the neurology appointment finally rolled around, he was feeling absolutely miserable. So while Alex screamed, the doctor examined him, more annoyed than ever and making no effort to hide it. When he finished, he looked at me and said, "He's autistic. And I'm telling you this at a great inconvenience to myself," and he walked out of the room. To this day, his voice still rings in my ears. He'd just told me that the life I'd always dreamed of—my life, Alex's life—was over. And off he went to his vacation.

I am not a believer in the "Holland versus Italy" story.[1] It has circulated for years on the Internet and it's always made me absolutely insane. It goes something like this: having a child with a disability is just like thinking you were going on vacation to Italy but finding out that instead, you've landed in Holland. Sure, Holland isn't the land of "the Coliseum, Michelangelo's David, the gondolas in Venice" that you were expecting, but it DOES have some lovely things too, like nice flowers, for instance. Yup, Holland's OK because it has nice flowers.

I can't speak for other childhood disabilities, but finding out your child is autistic is NOT like finding out that you've landed in Holland. For us, for Alex and me, the land of autism looks a whole lot like Dante's vision of hell: pain, pain, and more pain. So little sleep that you go insane: sickness, doctors, hour upon hour of high-pitched screaming, manic laughing, watching your child attack himself in his pain, blood, vomit...

If this is Holland, then I can't imagine it is one of the world's top ten tourist destinations.

For us, autism is Satan's realm. And when you enter, you're supposed to "Abandon all Hope," aren't you?

We were thrown into this world more than 11 years ago. Over these years we have tried treatment after treatment, from pharmaceutical medications to Chinese medicine, and therapy after therapy, from sensory integration to psychology. Time after time I have come ever so close to losing all hope. Hope, however, is my middle name and it's not in my nature to give up. I have always believed that out there, in this world, there are things that are going to help Alex.

I am determined to find every last one of them.

* * * *

Dr. Baker: *The awakening of hope and the power of intention that hope kindles are the fundamental tools of all who minister to our friends, patients, clients, parishioners, and congregants. Hope is the platform from which all other interventions attain the altitude where the strongest healing winds blow. Is there any discipline beyond the steep banks of mainstream "scientific" medicine where practitioners of the healing arts quench hope as a regular part of their early dialog with those who seek their help? Within mainstream medicine a deep, cold current lies in pediatrics, emerging from a bias that developmental problems lie beyond the reach of medical intervention. I believe that this bias predates the days of prescription pad medicine and must have roots that descend to archaic notions that lay at the boundaries of religion, superstition and medicine. As* *such intractable problems as cancer and mental illness in adults emerged as proper targets of biomedical and pharmaceutical intervention, pediatricians and pediatric neurologists carried into the 20th century a contrary way of thinking that gave an authoritative voice to the malignant words, "Don't look for answers." After an evaluation that may have consisted of anywhere from seven minutes of casual observation to three days of testing, these words continue to be uttered by experts in child care who finish off their assessment with a diagnostic label, advice on a behavioral/educational program, and the words, "Bring him back next year and let's see how he is doing." One hand on the doorknob, the expert may turn back to deflect the questions that pursue his or her escape from the exam room. "Hey, if you think you can find the cure for autism, you are just wasting your time and money and putting your kid through a lot of unnecessary expense and some serious risk."*

The fact is that parents who have looked for answers have found the causes of autism spectrum disorder (ASD). The causes have come to light as researchers pursued the implications of parents' reports of "what has worked for my child"—crucial data collected by Drs. Bernard Rimland and Steven Edelson of the Autism Research Institute since the 1960s (which was when Dr. Rimland's book Infantile Autism destroyed the myth that autism was caused by cold mothers). This book, to which Judy has invited me to add my perspective on the issues raised by the widespread success of SCD for children on the Autism spectrum (as well as children with many other vexing chronic illnesses), provides details about one strand in the web of information about "what has worked for my child." This web comes from the combined experience of parents—joined by practitioners and scientists—that has given us the current map of the landscape of ASD. Pioneers like Mary Coleman, M.D., and Gene Stubbs, Ph.D., created a body of evidence that predates the Defeat Autism Now! (DAN!) Network. Since the foundation of DAN! in 1994, practitioners, scientists, and parents benefit from their membership in a large family in which a strong collaborative spirit inspires our search for a common ground in which looking for answers is exactly what we are all about.

* * * *

By the time he was 15 months old, Alex had massive, continual, profound diarrhea pretty much every day of his life; every day that is, except those in which he was severely constipated. The constipation would eventually relieve itself in yet another torrent of liquid diarrhea. By the time he was two and a half, he was vomiting several times each week. If we were lucky, he would eat one meal a day. By this point we were at the doctor's office almost weekly.

It is a terrifying moment when you suddenly realize that our lauded Western medicine, which can pull one person's kidney out and stick it into someone else, which can mend hearts, reattach limbs, and separate twins attached at birth, is still in so primitive in so many ways.

The fact is that doctors cannot cure most things. They cannot cure any virus. That old joke about finding "a cure for the common cold" is no joke. They cannot cure any of the many known autoimmune diseases. In reality, most of modern medicine involves either finding ways to mask symptoms via the prescription pad or repairing body mechanics, using equipment and materials created for the doctors by engineers. If you have a cold, you take a cold remedy that does nothing to kill the virus itself but only makes your runny nose clear up. If you have allergies, you take Zyrtec or Allegra. You're still allergic but as long as you pay your dues to the pharmaceutical industry, you won't feel quite as awful. If you have depression, you can take Prozac. All the things that have made you feel depressed, whether they are psychological or physiological, are still there but you just don't care quite so much anymore.

If, however, the mechanics of your body are fouled up, if you need to have a valve in your heart fixed or a broken leg reset, THEN you're in luck.

The worst of all situations is when you don't have a name for your illness, because that irregular-polygon-shaped puzzle piece you've brought to your doctor does not have a corresponding insurance company hole to fit in. If you don't have an ICD 9 code, you're in BIG trouble.

I never realized this. Not until I brought my baby to the doctor because he was sick and was getting sicker.

* * * *

Dr. Baker: *The naming of your problem brings relief. Even if relief's companion, grief, comes with the deal, getting a label at least gives you the sense that "Well, at least they know what it is." The whole idea in medical practice as I learned it is to make a diagnosis and then base treatment on the collected evidence from the group of people who have that diagnosis. Prescribing treatment based on the diagnosis works very well for acute illnesses, because in*

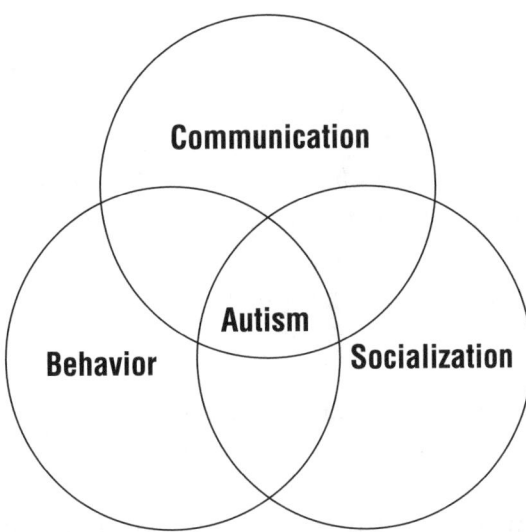

**Autism is an idea formed about groups of
children with three overlapping problems**

these cases the name tells us that what you see is what you've got—such as a splinter in your finger or pneumonia on an x-ray.

   Prescribing treatment based on the label of a chronic illness is a trickier business. Autism, for example, is a chronic illness in which the diagnostic criteria consist of three overlapping circles of evidence based entirely on observation of the patient. Autism is a name, or, properly speaking, it is an idea we form about a group of people. It is not the cause of anything—certainly not the symptoms. To say that symptoms of any sort are caused by autism is a trap of circularity into which many people fall whenever they open their mouths to explain what is happening to our kids. If you understand that autism is an idea, a notion, a convention of speaking that brings together three sets of observations about a group of individuals, then you will have a much easier time understanding everything Judy and I tell you in this book. Autism is not a thing, it does not attack people, and it is not the target of treatment. It is, most of all, not the end of thinking about your child. Getting a diagnostic label of any kind should never foreclose, but always open, thinking about what caused the illness and what is the first step in treatment for the individual (not the disease) in question.

   Notice that I said first step. When you are handed a diagnosis of autism you are likely to be simply overwhelmed with the whole situation, especially the biomedical options having to do with all sorts of things that your child might benefit from getting or avoiding. Judy and I will try to help you understand where SCD fits into the possible sequence of options for your particular child. Remember, however, that this is not rocket science. Mother Nature is very tolerant of flexible approaches because individuality was her idea and she does not expect perfection. She has a powerful inclination toward healing. Our job is to provide the conditions that help restore balance to vicious cycles so that they can be restored to the virtuous cycles from which they tumbled.

* * * *

What always amazes me about myself is that I say things that are true, and no one ever listens to me. Not even me, much of the time. I call this my Cassandra complex. (I often tell my family and friends that I'd like to change my middle name from Hope to Cassandra... and I have been *so* envious ever since I found out that one of my friends actually has this as her middle name.) Cassandra was a figure in Greek mythology who was cursed by the gods: she knew the truth but no one ever believed her. I said to our pediatrician, from the time Alex was just a couple of months old, that he was sick too often. I said that he wasn't like other babies: he was too hypersensitive and fragile. I said over and over that he was sick *all the time.* And how did she respond? "Well, what does he have?" Or else she'd explain to me that his bowel problems were due to his autism, as though autism were a germ—like a cold virus —that had the symptoms of diarrhea and vomiting.

The fact is, I was right. Alex was SICK, and this is what led to him developing autism. But even I didn't realize for years how sick he really was.

* * * *

Dr. Baker: *Alex was sick. Alex was sicker than most of the autistic kids I have ever treated. But all autistic kids are sick. It is just that some of them have findings that are more evident than others. If you look, the findings are there in all of them, if not in a careful history and physical exam, then in laboratory tests that reveal problems in three areas. The picture of how these three areas are interconnected is best grasped in a diagram that looks like the diagram of the old-fashioned diagnostic "communication, behavior, and socialization" criteria that are used to label kids as autistic. The similarity between the two diagrams is based solely on the need to show three related factors that can exist separately* but are equal to each other in importance when they occur together. In the case of the "oxidative stress, detoxification, inflammation" diagram we are dealing with "findings." These are features for which one has to look. This picture of the underlying pathology of autism did not emerge until the past few years because in the past there was a tendency not to look. Children with autism were judged to have a problem that was of psychological origin—cold mothers—until the 1960s. After that, most of the research money was spent chasing genetic factors, which turn out to play a role, but only in "filling the barrel," so to speak. It turns out that environmental toxins, antibiotics, viruses, and other factors burst the seams.

Alex's symptoms ranged and raged outside the neat circles of symptoms that gave him his label of autism. He was like many children whose picture includes a whole range of problems that have generally been unnoticed or ignored by physicians trained to discard details that are "unrelated" to the behavior, socialization, and communication problems needed to make the diagnosis upon which treatment options are determined. Alex's immune and digestive symptoms, and his persistent sallow pallor, the huge allergic shiners under his eyes, his failure to gain weight, and abnormalities revealed by laboratory profiles of his metabolism and immune system were exceptionally severe, but they exemplify the rule, not the exception, in ASD, where all affected children have features—if you look—of oxidative stress, inflammation, and problems in detoxification. The differences between autistic children and normal controls in these areas are huge.

In studies comparing one group of human beings to another, a difference of 15 or 20% is often enough to establish statistically significant differences that would, say, prove that a drug is effective or an environmental factor is noxious. Studies done over the past few years show us that autistic children differ by several fold in measurements of oxidative stress, inflammation, and detoxification. "Fold" doesn't come up very often in studies comparing different kinds of human beings. Let's look at one study to illustrate my point. Mark Blaxill, a parent and expert in data analysis, helped Amy Holmes, a physician, study the mercury content of hair taken from the first haircut—at around one year of age—from children who later became autistic and from those who later were normal. Parents cooperated by donating precious locks of baby hair that had been tucked away in their baby books. Children who became autistic had seven times less mercury in their baby hair than the normal controls. Seven times! That meant that these children had a very severe impairment in the detoxification chemistry needed to rid the body of mercury and other toxins. Jim Adams, Ph.D., has replicated the study and shown similar results. His analysis also shows a correlation of the mercury findings with the severity of autism.

Detoxification has to do with the body's ability to rid itself of substances that it doesn't want or no longer needs. That is, it deals with toxins normally found in plants, including the ones we eat as well as elementary poisons such as lead, mercury, etc., endogenous by-products (neurotransmitter, hormones, etc.), and toxins produced by gut flora that produce the odors familiar to anyone who has had a bowel movement or changed a diaper. These latter odors are particularly familiar to parents of the many autistic children who, like Alex, produce unbelievably foul-smelling stools and gas emblematic of something drastically unbalanced in the germs inhabiting their digestive tracts.

What about inflammation? A pimple is an example of inflammation. Redness, swelling, heat, and pain—these are the defining features of a process that medical students view under a microscope as a concerted effort of the cells of the immune system to cope with a foreign invader, whether it be a splinter or a virus. Since the days of my medical education, we've further refined the ability to observe inflammation by developing ways of measuring the chemicals that the cells of the immune system use to talk to each other. These molecules,

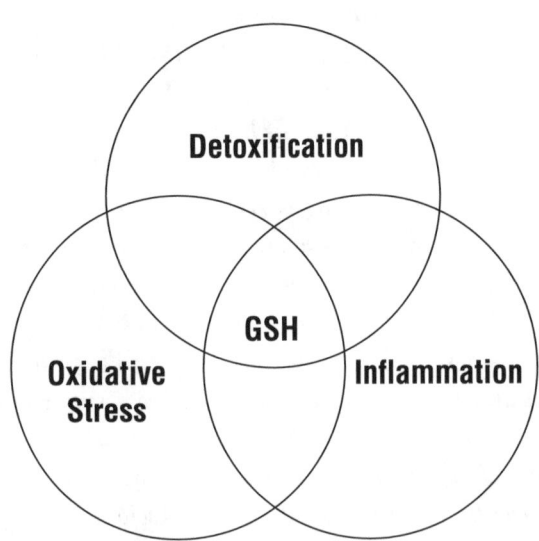

Glutathione is the main link in the chemistry of detoxification, oxidative stress, and inflammation

called cytokines, are made out of essential fatty acids found in vegetable and fish oils in our diet. When inflammation is present in a tissue, the immune cells shout to each other with cytokines, and tests for these molecules show very striking elevations in the tissues of autistic children as compared with normal kids. Again, we are talking about differences of many fold.

Oxidative stress? A burn, a sunburn, the heat of inflammation: these are manifestations of a process that is the very nature of fire itself. The flame of a candle results from oxygen (O_2) in the air stealing electrons from the molecules of wax. The lost electrons hook up with oxygen to turn it into water (H_2O). (That's right—there is water in the smoke from a fire. That's why you see a cloud of condensed water emerging from smoke stacks on a cold day.) The same kind of "fire" goes on in your body, where sugars and fats are oxidized at body temperature to get their heat for energy. This process also occurs when molecules other than oxygen try to bully our tissues' molecules into giving up electrons. Bullying molecules are often big ones such as heavy metals. Their oxidizing influence makes them sticky: when they cannot actually remove an electron from one of yours, they may "share" instead, thereby acting like fly-paper sharing its glue with the flies. Not good for the flies!

Jill James, Ph.D., has shown that autistic children differ markedly from normal controls with respect to measures of oxidative stress as reflected in levels of reduced glutathione (GSH). Notice that GSH is lies at the intersection of the three circles of the diagram. It is the link among them, and has evolved as a central factor in our understanding of the sickness of autism (I will return to this theme in my notes as we look at how SCD comes and goes in your child's treatment).

When Judy says that Alex was sick, she highlights the fact that doctors and others have, in the past, made a distinction between "having autism" and "being sick." What Alex shows us vividly and painfully is that autism is the sickness. And the sickness is autism. There is no boundary between autism's defining features of problems in communication, behavior, and socialization, its underlying features of oxidative stress, detoxification, and inflammation and its symptoms of pain, diarrhea, constipation, smelly poops, poor digestion, food sensitivities, rashes, headaches, fatigue, low muscle tone, and all the other manifestations of sickness that our kids display. It is a systemic problem of processing input from the environment, whether that input is words, pictures, sounds, touch, food, toxins, or the rhythms of life to which we all must keep in step. Failure to see sickness as a systems problem can only lead us back to a *primitive "name it and blame it and tame it—with drugs" approach that does not respect nature's impulse toward healing.*

* * * *

Alex couldn't communicate with me at all. When he was diagnosed he had the communication skills of a newborn: that is, he didn't even have a differentiated cry. I had no idea where the sickness was. He couldn't tell me. I began a search for a doctor who could help me sort it all out.

The first doctor we went to was a psychologist, or so he labeled himself. To this day, I'm quite convinced he actually meant psychopath and just got a little confused, what with the root word being the same and all. He asked us to leave the room while he "loosened Alex's sternum." You have to be wary of those tight sternums, he explained. In this case it was, he said, the source of Alex's autism. (No, I am not making this up.) When we refused to leave Alex alone with him, and started to stand up to leave— as one does when confronted with insanity—he held up a newspaper with a headline photo of the "Unabomber," who'd been caught that day, and said, "*This* is what he's going to grow up into if you don't take care of the problem now."

Of course, my first thought was, "Well, at least he'd be talking then!"

I spent the first four months after Alex's diagnosis finding an apartment in New York, moving us back from London, and then putting together our own home therapy team. The developmental pediatrician at Mount Sinai, who'd actually shown us some compassion when rendering his diagnosis, recommended that I take Alex to see a speech pathologist who'd help me get organized. I took Alex to see him the following week. The one worthwhile recommendation he made was to read Catherine Maurice's book, *Let Me Hear Your Voice*. She is a mother who cured her two autistic children via an educational methodology called applied behavior analysis, or ABA. In just seven months, her daughter was brought from silence, continual engagement in self-stimulatory behaviors, and many of the other symptoms of autism to fairly normal functioning.

I stayed up all night reading that book, four days after the diagnosis. By the morning, I knew that I could have Alex cured in less than seven months, because I knew I would work harder than anyone else in the world to fix him.

Recently, more than ten years after I had this thought, I was up all night with Alex. He never slept. Not one minute. He was so hyperactive he was positively twitching. So all night, we lay in his bed together so I could keep him quiet and prevent him from waking his brother. He still can't talk even enough to tell me what hurts. He has never shared with me a thought outside of expressing the most simple wants and needs. He can't read, write, dress himself, bathe himself, toilet himself....

I often regard myself as one of the greatest failures in the history of humankind. When I'm tired and worn out, on a cold, gray, rainy day, when I've been up all night and my eyes are burning and I can't get that lump out of my throat and I am wallowing in self-pity, I inwardly point a finger at myself and cry "LOSER!" But the truth is, in my heart of hearts, I know that's a lie. I could not have worked harder. Alex was just too sick. And the medical establishment had no help to offer us.

On May 8, 1996, about six weeks after the diagnosis, our first ABA therapist arrived at our apartment. "Call some other mothers," she recommended. "They know a lot that can help you." What was my first thought? "What could another mother know?" Even this many years later, I can't help but wince at the stupidity of that reaction.

Our therapist knew better. One day she refused to leave until I'd called another mother. I finally picked up the phone and the mom I spoke to gave me one of the best pieces of advice I've ever been given. "Go see Dr. Sidney Baker. Call today, because it can take awhile to get in to see him."

It took nine months or so, during which time Alex just kept getting worse, but we finally saw Sid Baker, and on that day our lives changed. Dr. Baker (a graduate of Yale undergraduate and medical school who has practiced pediatrics, family medicine, and finally, for many years, specialized in complex developmental illnesses like autism) is the coauthor of *Autism: Effective Biomedical Treatments*, or the DAN! manual, as it's commonly known.*

We all have those revelations when we realize that who we are today is in large part due to some formative moment in our past. For me, one of those moments was 2:00 in the afternoon, on March 8, 1997, when we walked into Sid's office. As if the very notion of having three hours to talk to a real live doctor weren't amazing enough, there was Sid's confirmation that I'd been right all along when I told people that Alex was physically sick and *that's* what was causing his autism. Then there was his knowledge of autism and his intellectual brilliance, which left us in awe. Finally, there was the way he looked at and talked about Alex, treating him as a human being and not a vegetable, which had us in tears for days afterwards. Dr. Baker showed us respect, gave us back our dignity, and offered us help with open arms.

I walked out of that meeting a changed person, with more new ideas and information than I'd ever gleaned in a three-hour period—and also, more hope.

I have told Sid that if there's one thing he does that will have the entire divine host out to fling open the gates of heaven for him, it's that he gives people hope. I would tell people that when we had an office visit with him, it was 50% for Alex and 50% for me. It was the fact that he was always thinking about Alex, always contemplating new information and new possible treatments that gave me that desperately needed boost every six weeks. I never left his office without regaining my spirits, my energy, my confidence, and my will to go on.

The main lesson I learned from Sid that first day was an entirely new concept to me. He told us that over the 30 years that he'd been practicing medicine, he'd learned the most from his patients. While it took me years to fully grasp the importance of that statement, I knew immediately that I was finally talking to a doctor who had some faith in me, who was actually listening to me and believed what I was saying. However, I didn't really "get it" for another six and a half years.

So, in March of 1997, Sid and I began a long and arduous journey together to look for a way to make Alex better. But nothing worked. Nothing. While other children made astounding progress right and left, Alex never made any progress at all. I spent years watching children get better, children start to talk, and children get mainstreamed into regular education classrooms, while Alex just got worse and worse and worse.

Alex's list of treatments with Sid is approximately 126 items long. The treatments range, literally, from A (alpha lipoic acid) to Z (Zyrtec).

* * * *

Dr. Baker: *From what vantage point did Judy watch children get better? Partly through my eyes, as I shared with her images of the improvement I routinely saw in other children. Partly through her friendships with other moms she met in her neighborhood and on the Web. She also became the host of an Internet bulletin board for a subset, (called the "Dr. Moms"), of moms and dads who* *formed what I called The Circle. This group was made up of parents I'd invited to social gatherings at DAN! meetings, friends she'd met along the way, and a network of people offering mutual support and information exchange by email and phone. It is safe to say that in the medical world in which I grew up physicians attached a certain negative value to communication among their patients. The waiting room could be seen and feared as a place where transmission of infectious ideas might upset the orderly transfer of information through the physician to the patient. In the world of my training there was an implicit hierarchy of authority with academic, governmental, and pharmaceutical voices at the top and the patient at the bottom. In this hierarchy, the physician served as a kind of funnel through which passed medical truth tailored to his or her patient's individual needs. The waiting room could be a place where comparison of how the doctor met individual needs. Now however, the explosion of support groups, books and magazine articles, and the access to information provided by the Internet over the past few decades, has upset the old pattern that followed a priestly role of the physician as the exclusive channel for medical truth.*

The movement that began with the publication of Dr. Rimland's book, Infantile Autism, turned the flow of truth about autism upside-down. The top-down system in which professors told doctors who told parents that autism was caused by cold mothers was flipped to become a bottom-up system in which Dr. Rimland and Dr. Edelson tabulated parents' answers to the questions, "What has worked for your child? What has given good results, bad results or had no impact?" My friendship with Dr. Rimland had many anchors, among which the firmest included a passion for letting the data talk and a solid belief in the reliability of the collective voices of parents. If there is any one principle that unites the members of the DAN! movement, it is a confidence in the value of listening to parents both individually and collectively.

Before I learned about SCD, my principal mechanism for "listening to parents" was the Autism Research Institute's periodic tabulation of the relative effectiveness—or lack thereof—of a long list of dietary, pharmaceutical, and nutritional interventions as reported in ARI's surveys. DAN! meetings were another important vehicle for communication. It was only after I learned about SCD that I began sponsoring social gatherings for my patients at DAN! meetings. Only after SCD did it finally occur to me to give all my patients the email addresses of the others for mutual support with yet another "impossible" diet and help in to coping with the practicalities of translating Elaine Gottschall's book into everyday life. When I started talking to my patients about SCD, I found that it took 40 minutes to just get parents to the point of even considering a diet that basically removed everything their kid was eating. Just as soon as I said, here's Judy's (or Jessica's or Heather's or Brenda's) email address and phone number, my problem was resolved. Other moms could not only sell the idea but provide the practical information needed to pull it off and the support required to get past the rough spots we see as the flora of the digestive tract adjusts to an upheaval in its ecology.

From then on, Judy's vantage point was enriched by regular, more formalized input from other parents who often saw prompt and relatively uncomplicated improvement in their kids while she, Judy, was in the trenches with Alex's SCD adventure. My own vantage point was elevated by being able to see through the eyes of a group of parents who were all starting SCD at more or less the same time, so that the periodic ups and downs that Judy describes became more evident than if the start times were random. SCD's appearance in my practice was the catalyst for turning my virtual waiting room into a big conversation among my patients by phone, email, and in person. This has enriched their resources and my own. Wherever you are, find other parents—preferably the ones who visit your doctor—because you will be spared some of the chaos of the unfiltered Internet, where you're less likely to find like-minded parents and more likely to find individuals pedaling products, war stories, fear, and the magnifications of small truths that are the downside of the Internet's wonderful access to information.

* * * *

But for Alex, all these things, which have helped so many other kids, did nothing. I spent my days mopping up body fluids. Constipation mixed with diarrhea. Diarrhea, diarrhea, and more diarrhea. Vomiting. I remember one day going upstairs to change my drenched clothing for the fifth time in a day and thinking: just a few years ago, I was a relatively attractive Wall Street broker with a big expense account. I drove my customers in limousines to the best restaurants in New York. I had friends, a social life, took vacations. And this is what my life is now. My life was defined by no sleep. Never any sleep. All day spent in vomit- and diarrhea-covered sweat pants.

What had happened to me?

One of the more repulsive symptoms Alex displayed was a stink. His body would reek, as I described it to Sid, "like a closed room with a thousand rotting carcasses in it." To get him out of bed in the morning I'd first fill up the bath with water and loads of fragrant soaps. Then I'd stand outside his door and take a deep breath, hold it, and run in to grab him and get him into the tub as fast as I humanly could. If I breathed before getting him in the water, I'd gag because the stench was so awful. Often, he'd have slept in vomit; although I'd usually be in his room the vast majority of the night, I'd sometimes miss the early morning vomit if he actually ever fell asleep and I finally was able to sneak back to my bed). But it wasn't just the smell of vomit. It was his whole body: the stink of putrification coming from *inside* him.

* * * *

Dr. Baker: *Stink. Of all the chronic illnesses that affect children, the one that is hardest on marriages is cystic fibrosis. I think it is the stink that does it as much as the oppression and trauma of a feeling of helplessness in the face of peril to one's child. Cystic fibrosis results from a failure of proper functioning of exocrine glands. As opposed to endocrine glands, which push their secretions of thyroid, adrenal, and gonadal hormones into the bloodstream, exocrine glands push their secretions onto the skin (sweat) and internal spaces of the respiratory and digestive tunnels of the body from the pancreas and mucous glands. Insufficient digestive enzymes cause a failure in the breakdown of dietary fat, carbohydrates, and protein so that food loses its nourishing capacity for the child and gains its nourishing capacity for the germs that inhabit the child's tunnels, with the consequence of lung infections and overgrowth of nasty germs in the digestive tract. Nasty equals stinky. Ninety percent of the germs that normally inhabit your digestive tract are anaerobic: that is, they thrive where there is no (an) air (aer) as opposed to being dependent on a supply of oxygen (aerobic). It is the anaerobic germs of the digestive tract that produce the normal unpleasant bathroom odors. When such germs are fed an abundant source of nitrogen and sulfur found in proteins, they can produce an absolutely overpowering stench that makes one feel an involuntary emotional need to flee the scene. I do not wish to trivialize the painful complexity of marital stress in a family with a chronically ill child. The problem clearly goes beyond olfaction. However, our sense of smell is so deeply connected to the emotional centers of our brain that we shouldn't minimize the importance of an urgent focus on the causative digestive problems of our kids.*

Autism is a digestive disorder in which the brain is downstream from bowel toxins. As I mentioned previously, the odors of normal stools tell us that the contents of the digestive tract are toxic. You would not want to live in a neighborhood that smells like that. Actually, human neighborhoods in regions of the world lacking public hygienic amenities do frequently have an odor that signifies to the approaching nose that humans live here, as surely as the odor of a barn and corral announce the presence of horses. In modern hygienic communities we have arranged to flush our poops and try not to live downwind of their destination, but we cannot avoid the transient escape of intestinal gasses in the toilet and, sometimes, in the parlor. It may be reassuring to know that you are not the author of the bad smells that come from your bowels (or breath or other body surfaces); rather, it is the germs that inhabit your body that should take the blame for antisocial behavior. Well-fed germs are particularly antisocial, as they are toxic to yourself and you can depend on the nastiness of the odor as a rough index of the toxicity. Recall that the stools of breastfed babies, whose digestion of their food is complete, have an odor that is not the least bit offensive. It is only with the introduction of non-human milk or other foods that babies' stools take on a normal smelliness produced by a more complex flora. When the flora become downright abnormal, then the odor becomes more powerful. When the flora's distribution becomes abnormal, with rising numbers in the normally relatively under-populated upper intestines, the potential for absorbing their toxins into the blood stream rises (with consequences that have not been explored very much in the medical sciences). One way or another—by its anatomical location or its internal balance among the 500 or so different species of bacteria and fungi—the gut represents an ecology as complex and as susceptible to damage as a Brazilian rain forest.

Medical tools for assessing the damage resulting from dietary imbalance, digestive failure, and antibiotics are very insensitive and our means for repairing and replacing damaged flora in some people are very imperfect. We do not understand why people differ in their ability to weather the storm of an antibiotic treatment without being bothered by yeast infections or other indicators of dysbiosis (abnormal numbers or distribution of intestinal germs). We do understand that if you stop eating altogether for a few days the flora die off and you stop producing bowel movements, which are composed of mostly germs, some undigested food fibers, and more or less water. A complete fast on nothing but water may have powerful healing influences for individuals with chronic illness. The various diets involved in the treatment of children with ASD are mostly efforts at partial fasting, in which the target of the fast is the flora, not the child. It is logical to ask whether antibiotics might be used to accomplish

the same result: getting rid of nasty gut germs. Indeed, the
especially in children in whom high levels of proprionate are
Proprionate (proprionic acid) is a compound made by gut ju...
shown by the research of Canadian scientist Derrick MacFabe to produce w...
effects in laboratory animals that look very much like the repetitive behaviors
of autistic children. Proprionate levels found in the urine of ASD children
can be reduced from 1,000 to zero in a few days of treatment with antibiotics
that kill clostridia, a group of especially stinky germs that predominate in the
gut flora. Transient improvement in symptoms has been reported in a group
of children treated with an anti-clostridia antibiotic (metronidazole) for six
weeks. Another treatment using oral gentamycin and vancomycin produces
odorless stools after a few days and symptomatic improvement in a very few
children. Generally speaking, however, antibiotic treatment does such damage
to normal flora that it just reproduces the very injury that may have initiated
the dysbiosis. Antifungal treatment is a different story, and is presented in detail
in Autism: Effective Biomedical Treatment (Drs. Sidney M. Baker and Jon
Pangborn).

* * * *

My babysitter used to help me wash Alex's sheets over and over to
try to get the stench out. Without exaggeration, sometimes it would take
five washings. The image of his sheets draped on the radiators around the
house (the dryer in that apartment never worked right) is one that still
comes into my head when I think about the bad old days.

Even worse for me is being flooded with images of so many days and
nights—in London, in New York, at my parents' house—spent walking
back and forth, back and forth, back and forth, trying to comfort and hold
Alex while he screamed hour after hour after hour after hour, back and
forth, back and forth, back and forth, and Alex screamed and screamed
and screamed, until his father and I were ready to kill ourselves or each
other.

Until you live it, you cannot understand what such a life is like. I
don't have the skill as a writer to convey the sense of time. I can't make
someone who hasn't been there understand what it is like: all those hours,
days, nights, months, years, of walking back and forth with Alex to try to
comfort him. All those years of not sleeping, until sleep becomes the most
valuable commodity in the house and you fight like animals over whose

.n it is to try to get your child to sleep, in the full knowledge that it's probably not going to happen and you're going to be up all night. You fight about who's going to get to take a nap and who's not. And it doesn't end. It just goes on and on and on and on...

Still, back then, as bad as things were I still had no real idea that it wasn't going to end. I believed in my own work ethic, I believed in Sid Baker, I believed in DAN! and Bernie Rimland—I believed I would be able to heal Alex. Perhaps it was a coping mechanism. To maintain sanity, you have to believe that things will get better someday.

That belief in a brighter future led us to talk about having another baby. I had always wanted more children and we thought that having a brother or sister would only help Alex. (At least in one thing we were right.) However, it was a hard decision. We consulted a geneticist. We had Alex examined and tested for any trace of known genetic disorders and when none were found, and our family history indicated no risk factors, we decided to fulfill our dream of a second child.

When Alex was almost three and a half, my younger son, Liam, was born. But things with Alex were not getting better and I was up with Liam, desperately trying to breastfeed him to save him from his brother's fate, while running in and out of Alex's bedroom night after night. Breastfeeding is commonly accepted by lay groups and medical and government organizations (such as the American Academy of Pediatrics and the USDA) as the healthiest way to feed a baby during the first year of life. Among its many benefits, breast milk provides infants with immunity to a host of diseases, colonizes the intestines with healthy flora, which are vital for proper digestion, and also keeps babies away from highly allergenic dairy and soy for longer periods of time.

* * * *

Dr. Baker: *Judy is perfectly correct in pointing out the support given to breastfeeding by the American Academy of Pediatrics and other authoritative bodies. It has not always been so. Nor is the support strong enough to combat the commercial interests promoting formulas, for which the recipes evolved from a pediatric art in the first decades of the 20th century. Pediatrics grew up as a medical specialty in a time when affluent families accepted the notion that bottle-feeding was "modern" and breastfeeding was a necessity only for the poor. Pediatricians touted the science of concocting formulas and would tweak* the recipe for combining water, cow's milk, and sugar every few weeks in ways that undermined mothers' confidence that they could manage the simple act of feeding a baby without technical know-how. Commercial interests seized the market created by this cultural and professional folly and have, ever since, promoted bottle-feeding against the interests of babies. Public policy, cultural sensibilities, employers of women, and families should support every effort to discourage the use of cow's milk or soy formulas and every measure that favors the feeding of human milk to human babies. Breast milk banks and wet nurses should be organized to expand every infant's access to nourishment that offers the best chance for creating the good brain and immune system needed for a healthy life.

* * * *

In August 1997, a little more than a month after Liam was born, we tried to take a vacation for a few days. We drove to the Hamptons, out on Long Island, and stayed in a rented house with my parents, my brother and his family. Alex's sleep was horrific and one night he went to sleep around 11:00, only to wake up at 12:00, screaming. The baby was sleeping and I was afraid that Alex would wake not only him but everyone else. So, in my pajamas, I put Alex into the car and for at least three hours drove around (and around and around and around…) the block, hoping and praying that the motion of the car would make Alex sleep, but it didn't work. I knew I needed to get back to feed Liam. I drove back to the house, grabbed Paul, the boys' father, and pushed him out to the car, and while I fed the baby, Paul drove Alex around and around and around…

He never went back to sleep that night.

In fact, he pretty much never went back to sleep.

One time, two months before Alex turned four, Paul went to the Super Bowl with his colleagues and Alex, Liam, and I went to my parents' home for the weekend. I'll never forget it. I'd finally gotten him to sleep around 3:00 or 4:00 in the morning and staggered into the bedroom next door. The next morning I went downstairs for breakfast, hearing nothing from his room and assuming he was still sleeping. Suddenly I heard a noise and ran up the steps. As I got about half way up, I smelled it. I called out to my Mom for help and opened the door to find the bedroom and Alex covered, absolutely covered, in diarrhea. The smell was like nothing I had ever smelled in my life, before or since. I ran into the bathroom and vomited.

My father ran around opening windows and spraying air freshener while my mother, gagging, grabbed Alex and put him into the tub. It took us a good hour to tackle the mess, gagging and vomiting, cleaning the diarrhea out of the cracks between the wood flooring with toothbrushes.

Alex was around four-and-a-half years old when I tried to take him to see a gastroenterologist. In the fall of 1998, I first saw Dr. Andrew Wakefield speak at a DAN! conference. For the first time, I started to have some idea of what had happened to Alex. I also realized, I mean really realized, that his bowel troubles weren't "because he was autistic," as we had been told over and over. They were real, and Alex wasn't the only autistic child to have the problem. Suddenly, I wasn't alone anymore.

Dr. Wakefield explained how he'd listened to the mother of an autistic child who claimed her son had terrible gastrointestinal illness. The mom told Dr. Wakefield that after her son received his MMR (measles/mumps/rubella) vaccine, he developed severe gastrointestinal symptoms, including vomiting and diarrhea. You can only imagine how I sat up in my chair, thinking, "Wait. That's ALEX she's describing. That's ALEX!" Dr. Wakefield arranged to have a colonoscopy performed on the child and he found that indeed his intestines were filled with ulcers and swollen, inflamed lymph tissue—generally agonizing pathology. When other parents told him that their children had regressed after the MMR shot, he committed the crime of believing them. He communicated his findings to other researchers with the skills and equipment to look for measles virus RNA in the swollen lymph tissue. Multiple different published studies have now confirmed Dr. Wakefield's original clinical findings. Also, the measles RNA has been isolated exactly where Dr. Wakefield said it existed.

His original paper was published in the illustrious British medical journal The Lancet, in February 1998. His conclusion reads, "We did not prove an association between measles, mumps, and rubella vaccine and the syndrome described [that is, the newly named "autistic enterocolitis"]. Virological studies are underway that may help to resolve this issue."[2]

Not long afterward, Dr. John O'Leary, of Trinity College, Dublin, did confirm the finding: "The data confirm an association between the presence of measles virus and gut pathology in children with developmental disorder."[3]

Dr. Wakefield's and Dr. O'Leary's findings caused explosive controversy in the medical establishment worldwide. Naturally, there were and are plenty of researchers and physicians who strongly dispute these findings. At this time, no one is really disputing that autistic children in this current epidemic are suffering from gastrointestinal and immune system disease. The question that is so hotly contested is: what is *causing* it? There is plenty of research on both sides of the argument. If I insert the search terms "measles" and "autism" into Google, I am provided with 169,000 entries. But this book is not about the scientific debate over whether the MMR vaccine caused a chronic measles infection in Alex's small intestine that led to his immune-compromised state, his severe gastrointestinal condition, and his autism. It's about what I've observed as a mother: Alex's continual diarrhea started shortly after his MMR, as did the regression into autism. It wasn't until around the year 2001 or so that I learned about the ethyl mercury in all those vaccines he'd had prior to that MMR. But that's another story.

* * * *

Dr. Baker: *You may have read in the press that the link between autism and the measles component of the measles, mumps, and rubella vaccine has been disproved. It is odd that such reports rely exclusively on epidemiologic evidence and fail to even mention the biological evidence comparing measles-associated findings in autistic children vs. normal children. In science, proof and disproof in questions like the association between measles vaccine virus and autism do not rest on epidemiologic studies. The scientists who try—too hard—to convince us otherwise know better. When scientists insist on epidemiologic "proof" that there is "no problem" we might suspect that they are trying to cover up the biological evidence, which is very persuasive of a link. The link, however, probably can't be explained by a simple question of a single arrow pointing from the MMR vaccine to the autism epidemic. There are several arrows—some with points at each end—and several elements in the story of the autism epidemic. The elements are not only the MMR vaccine but also the DTP and other immunizing agents. Moreover, the debate includes questions about the safety of giving many vaccines in the same visit to the doctor; the interaction between sickness, antibiotics, and the preservatives and other toxins found in vaccines; and the policy of re-immunizing children who are already immune based on previous immunization. None of these questions has ever been studied in ways that come within a mile of proving safety. Indeed, some of the studies, such as the first safety study of MMR vaccine, have shown evidence that the vaccine* *was not safe, but the evidence was hidden.*

Immunization is one of the best things in the medical tool kit. When I practiced in Africa (while working in clinics in different regions), where many children die from infectious diseases of childhood, I could tell where immunizations had been organized and where they had not; I can attest to the enormous value of shots against TB, diphtheria, tetanus, whooping cough, measles, and polio. Children should be immunized against such illnesses. The scientific community in charge of public policy regarding immunization has acted as if they were on the side of the angels—good people doing a good thing— and they became complacent, perhaps distracted by their ties to the companies that sell vaccines. They became negligent of their duty to compensate on safety issues for the fact that regulations governing proof of safety and efficacy of vaccines have been about as lax as those regarding conflicts of interest for those making public policy.

The key point in approaching the whole issue of immunization is that there is a natural difference between public and private policy. You are not in charge of immunizing all the kids in town—only your kids. Even in a perfect world the rules would not be the same for private and public policy, because some kids are completely covered by one shot of each vaccine and others will never get immunity no matter how many shots they get of a given vaccine. But if you go looking for an individualized vaccine policy from your normal, good pediatrician, you will probably be blown off. For more details, get Stephanie Cave's excellent book, What Your Doctor May Not Tell You About Children's Vaccinations.

* * * *

Galvanized by Dr. Wakefield's findings, I made an appointment at Mount Sinai hospital with a gastroenterologist I'd seen speak at a conference on autism. I thought that with her interest in autism, she'd know about the paper Dr. Wakefield had just published and would be able to help Alex and me. She knew about the paper, all right. "He's a quack," she told me. "I won't scope your son. He has diarrhea because he's autistic."

First, we started Alex's life with antibiotics. Then, we administered mercury-laden vaccine after vaccine. Then came the MMR, which I believe was the proverbial straw on the camel's back.

The Defeat Autism Now! team holds to the following hypothesis laid out here by Dr. Baker, when he discusses Alex's history in the 2005 book *Autism: Effective Biomedical Treatments*:

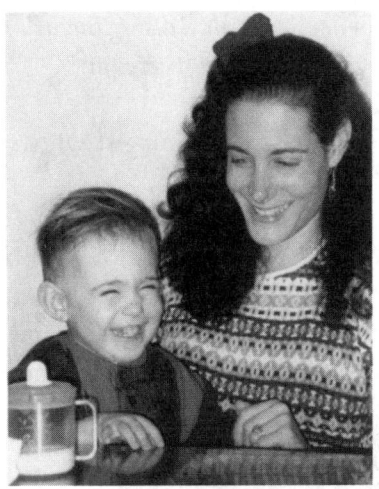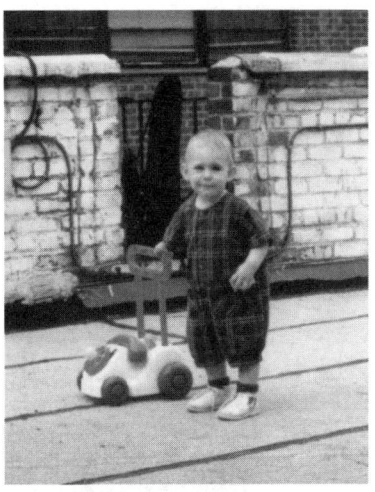

Normally developing Alex, around one year old

Antibiotics given in the first months of life increase the toxicity of mercury, and the combined effect of mercury toxicity and altered intestinal flora [the normal bacteria that inhabit the large intestine, that are critical for proper digestion] causes damage to Alex's digestive system, including a branch of his immune system that deals with the digestive system. This branch, the gut associated lymphoid tissue (GALT), constitutes the biggest and busiest part of the immune system. As a result, he may be more susceptible to both typical and atypical infections.... Injury to the gut is associated with symptoms such as diarrhea, constipation, and difficulty with digestion. Difficulties with digestion permit the incomplete breakdown of certain proteins.... Products of this incomplete digestion enter the bloodstream by way of Alex's damaged gut, which is abnormally permeable to these products.

When he is administered a vaccine combining three live viruses (mumps, measles and German measles—the MMR), Alex's immune system is unable to rid his body of the live measles vaccine virus, which instead of being transiently present in saliva, persists in his body where it can be found months or years later in his GALT as well as in his spinal fluid...

At some point in this progression, Alex begins to display symptoms related to toxicity and dysfunction of his central nervous system, and *slowly or abruptly passes into a state of developmental disorganization which leads doctors to give him a label on the autism spectrum."*[4]

It took me another four years to find a gastroenterologist who would look at Alex. When he did, we knew the truth.

Meanwhile, I began to observe the first self-abusive behaviors by Alex when he was six years old. It all started with what we called "finger bending." Alex would pull his pinkies over the back of his hands, to a 90-degree angle eventually, as the ligaments stretched. Then he started to bite his lips until they bled. By the time he was seven, he was scratching himself to

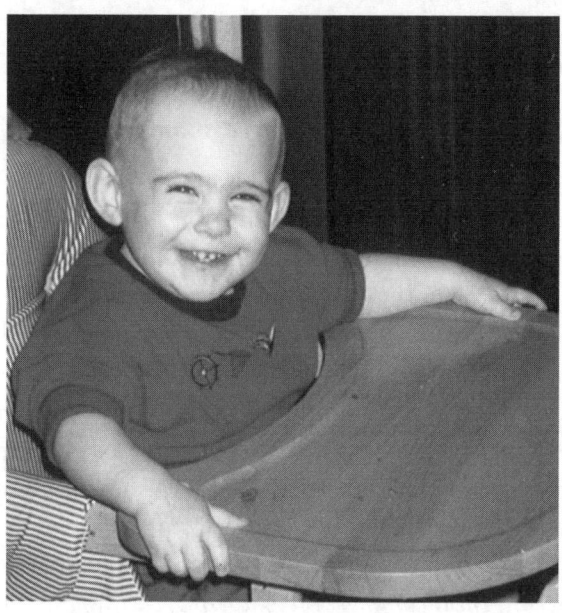

Here is a picture of Alex on his first birthday, March 3, 1995

the point of drawing blood. Then, the "body banging" started. Alex would crouch next to a coffee table or another hard piece of furniture and whack his arms and body into it as hard as he could.

All through these years, he was making no progress in terms of language, cognition, academic skills, or social skills.

I believe that for a parent of a sick child, there's no day of the year worse than your baby's birthday. Another year gone—another year in which you've failed to help. Another year of unbearable suffering passed. And you're his mother. You're supposed to make things better, but you can't. We "celebrated" birthday after birthday, putting a cake in front of Alex that he didn't care about, giving him presents he had no interest in…

I can't finish typing that paragraph. It hurts too much.

By the time Alex was eight, our situation had become dire. In the summer of 2002, he began to break things. It started with small objects, like cordless telephones and remote controls. We lost countless numbers of remote controls, telephones, lamps, and answering machines. If we left one of these in his sight for even a few seconds, it was destroyed. Every time we would lose something, everyone in the house would be at each other's

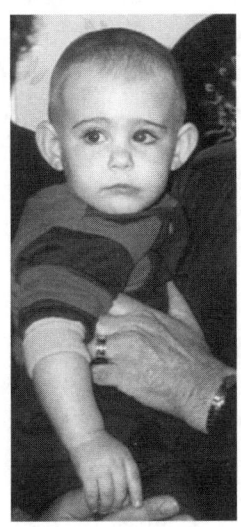

Here he is, ten days later, four days after his MMR vaccination

throats, yelling accusingly, "Why'd you leave it out?" Then the behavior escalated. Alex began to smash our TVs, computers, pictures, and furniture.

Another of my least favorite memories: sitting at the breakfast table and suddenly hearing a monstrous crash from the next room. We ran in to find Alex standing over the remains of our 40-inch color television. Then there was the time we were upstairs in Liam's room. Before we even registered what he was doing, Alex had pulled down Liam's seven-foot wooden bookcase, almost killing himself in the process. Then there was the time I woke to a thunderous crash from Alex's room and found that he'd pulled over his lamp. There were bits of glass from the cracked bulb everywhere, with Alex standing over the mess in his bare feet. There were also the heart-stopping crashes coming one day from the basement, where I found him standing amid piles of glass as he ripped all the pictures off the walls and threw them. Not a day went by when we didn't lose something. At the worst times, I would have to take Alex into the bathroom with me and hold on to him while I used the toilet. It wasn't just that he couldn't be left alone for even a minute; it was that he literally had to be held onto every second he was awake. Let go of him, to cook, bathe, pick up the phone, use the toilet, etc., and something was in pieces.

Alex isn't really verbal, so he couldn't tell me what was going on. But I knew in my heart that he was smashing things because he was in unbearable agony—and nothing I tried ever made it better.

When I was about 21 years old, I learned a very valuable lesson from my hamster, Herman. I was going through a rough time emotionally, still depressed over the death of my very much loved grandfather, and lost, because I'd graduated from college before I was ready and still didn't know what I wanted to be when I grew up. One particularly awful morning I sat in my apartment crying before heading off for work. I looked up at my flat mate and exclaimed in despair, "What else could go wrong?!" I stood up and went to feed Herman, only to find him dead.

I learned at that moment that something else can always go wrong. And with Alex, it did.

There was the time he was beating himself against the furniture in the den. It took both Paul and me holding him on the floor to keep him from killing himself. I *almost* thought, "Nothing else can go wrong. This is the worst it can be," when suddenly the telephone rang. It was my grandmother's assisted living facility calling to tell me (since my parents were in Italy and my aunt was in North Carolina) that they'd had to bring her to the emergency room and could I come.

We were desperate. Absolutely, positively, 100% desperate.

In November of 2002, four months before Alex's ninth birthday, I finally got a look at the source of Alex's eternal pain. Sid got us an appointment with a gastroenterologist who brought Alex in for a colonoscopy the very next day. Here are pictures of what my son had been living with every day for at least seven years. The truth was that Alex had colitis, cryptitis, and lymphoid nodular hyperplasia. The truth is, had he not been autistic, the medical establishment would have found this out and treated it seven years before.

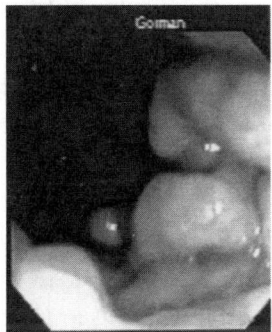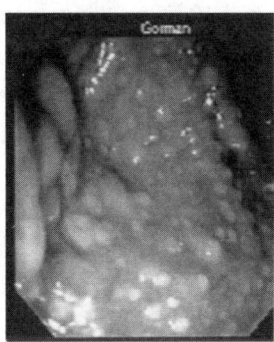

The lining of Alex's intestine: the swollen lymph tissue is readily visible

What do colitis, cryptitis, and lymphoid nodular hyperplasia mean? Technically, it means that his intestines were severely inflamed, ulcerated, filled with large, inflamed nodules (pockets). You can see these clearly in the photos above. It also means that the mucus crypts of his intestines, which normally allow food substances and bowel movements to pass painlessly through the intestines, were infected so that there was no protective coating on Alex's already-inflamed intestinal lining. Functionally, it means that he was in agony for almost all of his life. It also means that everything he ate was improperly digested (so that he absorbed little, if any, nutrients from his food), and that undigested food could leak through the ulcerations in the intestines directly into his blood stream, causing immune system havoc and acting as false neurotransmitters, thereby sending false signals to his brain.

Finally, I had seen the enemy. Naively, I believed that now, having demystified it, I would be able to conquer it. I thought that this time, this time finally, we knew what we were fighting and could beat it.

As always, Sid, our gastroenterologist, our immunologist, and I tried many therapies to heal Alex's intestines, but as always, things only got worse.

****

Dr. Baker: *The medical priesthood's special status depends on its capacity to see, and name, the often invisible, sometimes useful manifestations of illness. X-rays and other imaging studies, biopsies, cultures, and tests of allergic, immune, and biochemical factors allow us to "see the enemy" when a bone fracture, a specific causative germ, or a signature chemical abnormality—such as a very elevated blood sugar level or very low serum ferritin—points to the cause of pain and swelling in an arm, a bad sore throat, thirst and frequent urination, or iron-deficiency anemia.*

I say "sometimes useful" because naming and blaming often merely create the illusion that we have the power to tame a problem. Making something visible by giving it a name is especially reassuring when it gives us the sense that "the doctor knows what I've got." It is an illusion when, as in the case of most chronic illnesses, we are given the name of a group of people who share certain features, or the name of a kind of inflammation, when the name doesn't lead to a specific treatment such as iron for iron deficiency. The red, hot, swollen, painful tissue in Alex's digestive tract had not been silent—as it may be in many autistic children—but had been announcing its presence with symptoms of stinky diarrhea and abdominal pain that were more than sufficient to say he had inflammation of the bowel. Actually laying eyes on that inflammation was enormously reassuring to Judy and was part of a discovery process that unfolded when three prominent gastroenterology specialists (Drs. Andrew Wakefield, Tim Buie, and Arthur Krigsman) became regular contributors to the DAN! movement, bringing their diagnostic tools to the task of understanding autism in a new light: the light at the end of their endoscopes.

The date on the pictures of Alex's intestinal lining is 11/20/2002. By the fall of 2006, the DAN! consensus recognized that autism is more usefully understood as a bowel problem in which the central nervous system is downstream from the gut than as a brain problem in which the gut is "involved." Let's remember that autism, like all chronic illnesses, is a systems problem in which everything is interconnected so that simple linear cause-and-effect thinking is less useful in deciding what to do than respectful attention to multiple factors. Still, deciding what to do always demands a sense of priority. From the time of the first DAN! meeting in 1995, there has been a strong consensus among us that dealing with the gut issues takes first priority in the clinical approach to children with autism. As our gastroenterologist colleagues have brought their insights, "dealing with the gut issues" has bifurcated. One fork in the road leads to concerns about the roles of diet and flora in causing or perpetuating the vicious cycles of inflammation. The other fork is the more medically mainstream effort to suppress inflammation with steroids and other anti-inflammatory drugs. Each approach has its merits; the individual child is the expert in deciding which approach produces the best lasting results for him or her.

We all shared Judy's naïveté in thinking we had found the answer as more and more endoscopies and colonoscopies revealed the nearly universal severity of gut inflammation in autistic children. Subsequent scientific studies, comparing large groups of children with autism to children with other inflammatory bowel problems and to normal children, reveal that nearly all autistic children have unique differences in the cellular and biochemical (cytokine) patterns of their inflammation. The differences between the autistic and other children are many fold, making them as utterly recognizable as is that of the behavior of a severely autistic child caught in a moment of distracted stimming or a meltdown. If, as Judy implies, we were inside-out, so that the troubles of our intestinal mucous membrane were as public as our facial skin, autism would have been known for years as a bad bowel rash with associated behaviors and not the other way around.

* * * *

In September of 2003, we hit rock bottom. Alex was having 15 or more bowel movements a day. He was vomiting multiple times each week. One day in particular stands out in my mind. I was trying to get the boys up and ready for their school buses. Since he was five years old, Alex has gone to special schools for children with severe autism. I went down into the basement, which by then was pretty well Alex-proofed in that everything that could be smashed already was, and found him down there having plastered everything with bright yellow vomit.

His constant nausea made every meal a battle. He was drastically underweight. He was learning nothing. He spent most of his school day in the bathroom and when he wasn't at the toilet, he just ran around the classroom looking for things to smash. We couldn't go anywhere, we couldn't do anything. And all this while he was on the medications Prednisone, Colazol, 6MP, Nexium, and Gastrocrom.

Then one late September day I got a phone call from our gastroenterologist, who said that we had to take Alex off Prednisone. He'd been on so much that it was getting dangerous. Large doses of steroids, taken over long periods of time, put patients at risk for developing steroid psychosis—that is, an insanity whose symptoms include "emotional lability, anxiety, distractibility, pressured speech, sensory flooding, insomnia, depression, perplexity, agitation, auditory and visual hallucinations, intermittent memory impairment, mutism, disturbances of body image, delusions, apathy, and hypomania."[5] Now, if you can imagine a severely autistic child developing hallucinations and delusions, you can understand that it's probably better to avoid steroid psychosis...

At least the Prednisone had controlled the worst of Alex's pain. The prospect of going off it was unbearable. Worse, the doctor wanted me to put Alex on something called an "elemental diet": that is, no more food, only a liquid nutritional supplement. I couldn't do that, not to my boy. It's not that Alex loved eating by any stretch of the imagination. But on better days, he still loved chips, French fries, pretzels, dry cereal. And with so few enjoyments in his life, the thought of taking those few precious things away from him was just horrible. "I can't believe this is the best I can do for Alex. I can't believe this is the only answer." This is the supreme agony: looking at your suffering child and knowing that you are absolutely helpless, absolutely powerless, to make it better.

* * * *

Dr. Baker: *Was there actually something Judy could not do to help sort out Alex's problem? She was already far beyond the limits of what most mothers or fathers are asked by their child's illness. Normal—that is average—parents of autistic children often draw the line at anything beyond drugs and ABA. Their pediatricians and other specialists have said, "Don't look for answers." They wait patiently for the promises of genetic research or for the results of a trial of another psychotropic drug. That's what normal people do. The parents who look for answers are exceptional in their capacity to swim against the tide of opinion that says that the answers come from above—from the scientists, the government, the drug companies—and that looking for them to come from one's own experience is foolish at best and dangerous at worst. Only one of the hundreds of sets of parents I have known has not been rewarded by their efforts to find biomedical answers for their autistic child. Benefits of biomedical treatment justify their intellectual, emotional, and financial costs more than 99% of the time. Judy had gone the distance. She had seen only one brief flicker of improvement at the beginning of Alex's treatment with me. She'd encountered* *failure with treatments that were, let's say, less extreme than an elemental diet (in which a complete recipe of basic nutrients—sugars, amino acids, fatty acids, minerals, and vitamins—is given as a formula that requires no digestion and is presumed to have no capacity to evoke an allergic response). Why would she balk at that? Because the formula was loaded with sugar and it was to be administered via a percutaneous endoscopic gastrostomy (PEG), which is a tube passed into the stomach through a hole created in the abdominal wall. That was just too much—not so much because of the hole as because she knew that the sugar would make him worse. That thought triggered her memory of the no-sugar diet she had heard about.*

I had been reminded of the SCD a week or so before Judy asked me about it, and I was ready to say "Go for it." Recalling that I had heard of Elaine Gottschall's work and book several years before from my friend, Dr. Leo Galland, I called him and got a thumbs up on using it for patients with inflammatory bowel disease. I was ashamed for not having latched onto it when he had first mentioned it to me, but it just didn't stand out on my radar screen. I was already up to my ears in allergy elimination diets, yeast-free diets, high-protein diets, high-fiber diets, low-fat diets, casein-free diets, gluten-free diets, and Feingold diets, and just had too much on my plate at the time. In the 1990s I was, moreover, still thinking of autism as a central nervous system problem often accompanied by bowel disease rather than the other way around.

* * * *

As I write this book, it has been more than 11 years since Alex was diagnosed. I have looked for ways to help him every one of those days. It took me seven and a half years to find the first thing.

But find it I did.

And it wasn't a doctor who helped me to find it.

September 2003: "Take Alex off Prednisone. Put him on the elemental diet."

Something in me snapped. I sat at my desk—right where I'm sitting now, three-plus years later—and thought that the time had come for me to take Alex and jump off a bridge. I sat at my desk picturing the moment of death, contemplating the best way to end this torture. It would put Alex out of his agony—and because I can't live without him, it would put me out of mine.

But at that worst possible moment, I remembered something I hadn't thought of in years. I remembered meeting another mom at a DAN! conference. I was looking through some books on diet and she interrupted my perusal to tell me that I should buy a book called *Breaking the Vicious Cycle* be-

> *Some people hope for a miracle cure,*
> *Some people just accept the world as it is.*
> *I'm not willing to lay down and die...*
> – Billy Joel, "An Innocent Man"

cause her really sick son was doing fantastically on the diet described in this book. I'd bought it at the time but had forgotten about it, what with the 800 other things on my immediate list of things to do back then.

I'll never know what made me suddenly think of that mother and that book, but I pulled it off my shelf and started to read. By the time I'd finished the third chapter, I knew that this was the diet for Alex. *Breaking the Vicious Cycle* lays out the particulars of a diet called the Specific Carbohydrate Diet, whose basic premise is the removal of all complex carbohydrates from the list of allowed foods. More on this later. I started Alex on SCD at dinner that night.

At the end of three months or so on SCD, Alex went down to five or six bowel movements a day, and they were slowly becoming more and more formed. I gradually dared to take him off medication after medication. By the time he was on the diet for four or five months, he was off all gut medications and was down to two or three bowel movements a day. As soon as I'd started the diet, he'd immediately stopped all vomiting and had begun to eat at least one meal a day, sometimes even two or three.

Now, as I write this, he has one to two formed bowel movements each day almost all the time. He has vomited only three times since being on this diet. When Alex was three, we discovered that his immune system was so dysfunctional that he required gamma globulin IVs to live. Gamma globulin is purified human antibodies that are delivered intravenously. Each IV treatment takes four or five hours to deliver. Alex had been started on this treatment just after his third birthday. Every three weeks (sometimes every week), for seven years, we'd take him to the doctor for his gamma globulin IV. After six months on SCD, he was able to stop getting the treatment, and he has been sick no more often than is normal. He has gained more than 30 pounds since starting SCD and is now in the fiftieth percentile in both height and weight.

* * * *

Dr. Baker: *Globulins are a family of proteins with a globular (round) as opposed to a stringy, shape. Antibodies are sticky globular proteins that adhere to and deactivate foreign materials that come into the body. Antibodies stick so specifically to their target substances that they are effectively a system for labeling everything that you come into contact with in your life. They are the basis for your immune system's primary role as a memory of your experience of the world of tiny things, just as your brain contains the memory of your experience of the big world of seeing, hearing, and other senses. Together, your immune system and your central nervous system remember, recognize, and organize your picture of the world so that you can respond to it appropriately.*

The chemistry of autistic individuals is disorganized in ways that present them with a distorted picture of the world at the immunological and sensory levels. The disorganization of immune chemistry is not represented by a limited set of abnormal lab tests. On the contrary, in different individuals and to different degrees, the disorganization is expressed in ways that can be measured in dozens of different lab test abnormalities. To understand this disorganization, picture a seesaw where one end is represented by TH1 (thymus helper cell type one) and the other by TH2 immunity. TH1 has to do with three very different targets—cancer cells, viruses, and fungi—that share one feature: you never met a friendly one. TH2 immunity has to do with making antibodies to everything else, including your own tissues (autoimmunity). TH2 immunity requires decisions about friends vs. foes on a regular basis and tends to work overtime in autistic individuals. That is, ASD children tend to have their seesaw tilted with the TH1 end down and TH2 up.

Why, then, does it work to give antibodies as intravenous gamma globulin (IVGG) (or immune globulins, IVIG)? IVIG supplies antibodies for people who fail to make enough for their own protection, and it blocks auto-antibodies. Both factors appear to result in problems for autistic individuals who, for example, may fail to have an appropriate antibody response after various immunizations or may produce overabundant antibodies against foods, inhalants, germs, or their own tissues (such as a brain protein called myelin basic protein). Immunological strategies for individuals with autism are beneficial when they help increase TH1 and decrease TH2 immunity. Alex had measurably low blood levels of gamma globulin that were picked up on a screening blood test that is routine in infants who have recurring infections or fail to thrive. Thus, he qualified for IVIG treatment quite apart from its possible cognitive or behavioral benefits. Deficiencies of blood globulins and recurring infections are criteria that insurance companies use for reimbursement for IVIG, which is costly. Children with normal serum globulin levels have benefited from IVIG. In them, the benefit may come from blocking auto-antibodies or in providing specific help against chronic infection with viruses or fungi.

* * * *

On top of that, because Alex can now sit comfortably, we're able to start teaching him again. I know it may sound a little silly to write about how thrilled I am that Alex is, for the first time in his life, saying yes and no, considering that he is 13 now and this is a one-year-old skill. But to me, this is not silly at all. It's a sign of the first progress he has ever made.

We have even gone on several vacations because now I can take him on airplanes. Two summers ago I took Alex to England and Greece for a full two-week holiday in Europe.

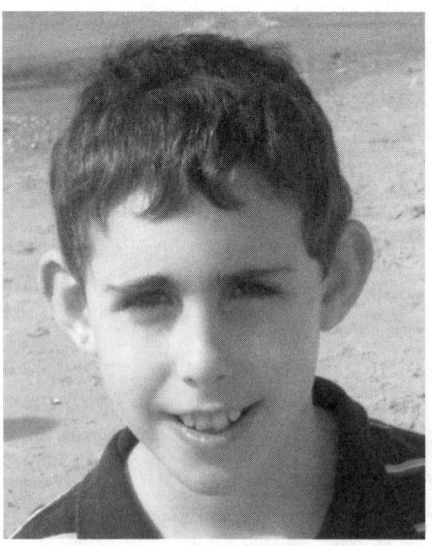

On the beach in France

My son is 13 and still profoundly autistic and still very, very sick. Some might say that I've failed. There are some days I feel I can't do this anymore. I can't bear the knowledge that I am failing, over and over and over.

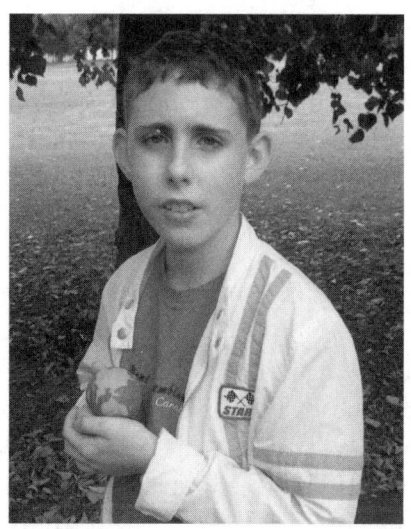

Playing ball in a London Park

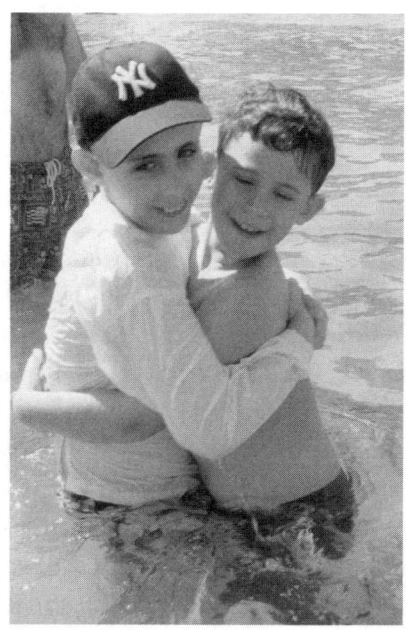

My boys playing together in the Ionian Sea,
at the beach in Corfu, Greece

I have tried so hard—as hard as I could—and look where we still are. But the truth is, I'm never going to give up. I've found one thing that works in SCD and I'm going to find more. I will do whatever it takes.

Most important of all, Alex no longer suffers the way he did for the first 12 years of his life. Often now, his is smiling and happy to be alive.

The Specific Carbohydrate Diet. The only thing I've ever done right for Alex.

Maybe I should think of it, instead, as the *first* thing I've done right for Alex.

I often use the following image to explain to my friends and new parents (that is, parents whose children have recently been diagnosed with autism, or parents who are just starting out with medical treatments for their children with autism) how I think about things:

The "cure" is somewhere up there in the heavens. For me to climb up to it, as it is extremely far away in Alex's case, I need to build a very stable structure. Geometrically speaking, the most stable of all structures is the pyramid. So, I need to build a very solid pyramid, stone by stone (treatment by treatment), to reach that cure. Every child's cure-pyramid is going to look different, based on individual biochemistry, but without the most solid and stable of bases—a working, healthy digestive system—the stones I try to use will have nothing to rest upon to keep them sturdy. SCD is that base.

* * * *

Dr. Baker: *Two of the meanings of "individual" have a clinical bearing on every way we think and everything we do. Individual means whole, or not divisible, and it means distinct by virtue of having a distinctive complexity. In a medical world in which diseases are seen as the target of therapy and people are paralyzed from useful thinking by statements that "there is no treatment for autism," it is particularly important to keep two points in mind. One is that the complex unity of each child's being means that it is seldom appropriate to single out a particular symptom as the target for a particular treatment, in the way that we would pick aspirin for a headache. Granted, that symptoms such as pain, too much or too little focus, insomnia, constipation, or hyperactive or repetitive behaviors may appear to yield to specific medications or supplements or diets. But usually it works best to view the whole child, and the balance of all the systems within that child, as the target of therapy and the basis for* the healing that nature provides when balance is achieved. Our choices work better the more we view the problem as a systems problem, in which everything is connected to everything else, and the less we see things in terms of linear causation, in which symptoms are isolated targets of different interventions.

The other point is that each child is unique. There is no one-size-fits-all approach to understanding and treating our kids. That aspect of individuality requires especially vigilant attention. Why? Because the trend toward the naming-blaming-taming that characterizes prescription-pad medicine drags us out of reality into a fantasy world where we speak of the symptoms caused by autism as if autism were a thing. Autism doesn't cause symptoms; autism is the name we give to a cluster of symptoms having to do with behavior, socialization, and communication. That cluster was named long before its biomedical causes were understood. In fact, it was named when its causes were completely misunderstood! Even today, when the biomedical picture of autism is grasped by some physicians, parents, and researchers, we have to beware of the legacy that comes with thinking about "What is the right treatment for autism?" instead of focusing on what is the right next step for this one child. When it comes to making the decision about what is the next step for a given child, keep in mind the distinction between a diagnostic test and a treatment. There may be a confusing overlap between the two, because most treatments in medicine really are tests to see if the treatment works. We err if we make a sharp distinction between sending blood or urine to the lab or making careful observation of how a child addresses certain tasks on the one hand, and giving a pill, prescribing a diet, or teaching in certain ways on the other. The pill, the diet, and the teaching are, at the outset, nearly always tests that should be viewed with an open tentative mind that says, "This child is the expert. He will tell us if this is the right approach. Let us look and listen respectfully to what this trial reveals before considering that it is the best choice." Trial and error? You bet. If someone says, "Just listen to me, I'm the doctor. I know best," think twice. First, think, "Are we talking about what is the preferred next diagnostic step?" Then think, "What are the other options, and at what point may we consider them?" If we understand that each child is a complex system, we can appreciate that our job has more to do with weighing options about the next step and committing to it only when we see a kid's response than it has to do with declaring that we know just what to do.

Having said these things about individuality, how do we have a useful map to guide us past the many forks in the path of decisions? One is to keep in mind that at each fork we can return to the two fundamental questions that define our basic strategy: **Is there something for which this child has an unmet need, which, if met, would help rebalance his system?** And, **Is there some toxin or allergen for which this child has a special intolerance and which he or she should avoid or be rid of?** Those two questions apply to everyone with a chronic illness.

Are there other general clinical rules that embrace all of our kids no matter how they may differ from others? Yes. There is one about timing and another about food. Timing is not an individual matter. In matters of biochemistry each of us is unique. In matters of timing, we all dance to the same beat—or, at least, we fail to do so at the peril of our health. Think of an orchestra or a band or a quartet or even a single voice or instrument producing a single piece of music. The way the sounds mesh has to do with whether it works as a whole or not. It is either in synch or out of synch. It is either in tune or out of tune. We can feel and hear the tuning and synchrony with the same precision with which we can spot, in a march of hundreds, the single person who is out of step. The rules of timing are very strict and there is a right and a wrong way—not a range of normal—to achieve harmony when rhythms are joined. Who is the conductor for the dance we all join, and in which our autistic children are out of synch? The simple answer is the day-night cycle of our planet. It is the same for all of us, and its imperatives have to do with sleeping, growing, detoxifying, and repairing at night, and eating, pooping, and doing the tasks of conscious living during the day. The big scale of the day-night (circadian) cycle is where many of our kids fail, with insomnia at night and impaired consciousness during the day. On the smaller scale in which our children's movements fail to synchronize with others around them we can feel and sometimes observe their lack of inner harmony and outer integration with their environment.

This is not the place for a full treatment of a complex subject, about which I have written elsewhere (The Circadian Prescription, Putnam, 2000) but it is a good place to introduce a key notion about food. It is not just that daytime is the time for eating and night is the time for sleeping and that is the way it is intended for all of us. It is also that morning is the better time to consume the larger portion of one's daily protein needs and evening is the time when carbohydrates should dominate. Of all the factors of timing that favor a healthy meshing of food supply with metabolic needs, the protein in the AM and carbohydrate in the PM emphasis is the one that is most relevant to our intentions to help our kids get into synch. Naturally, this consideration is pertinent to the subject at hand, SCD, because it tends to get us to restrict carbohydrates and automatically increase dietary fat and protein.

SCD's implications when it comes to the balance of protein, fat, and carbohydrate leads us from another way in which individuality is secondary on a very practical level to ways in which we are all similar. That is, none of us needs as much protein as those of us who have learned about nutrition over recent decades have been taught to believe. Plant protein is, moreover, good for us as compared with animal protein (fish, eggs, milk, and meat). The notion that plant protein is incomplete and nutritionally inferior is, in its essence, wrong. The notion that fish, eggs, milk, and meat are not only good for us but essential to a "well-balanced diet" is wrong. The evidence to support what I am saying is utterly persuasive but the combined effects of long-held beliefs, self-promotion of the food industry, and our acquired tastes and habits make it a hard sell. I can do no better here than to refer you to The China Study by the eminent scientist Colin Campbell, Ph.D. It is a book that reports the results and implications of a body of research that would, if acted upon, change the course of civilization by drastically reducing the toll of the chronic illnesses that characterize modern affluent societies: cardiovascular disease, cancer, the dementias of aging and the learning and behavioral problems of the young, diabetes, autoimmune disorders, and autism. The take-home message that underlies the claim that a plant-based diet would eliminate these problems is that they all share the same underlying landscape of interconnected features of oxidative stress, inflammation, and problems in detoxification. **Dietary remedies directed at this triad are not just another fad but a direct response to the need to address the common factors of diseases, in which all particular diseases arise with different names and symptoms depending on our genetic makeup.**

In summary, we are each different. The treatment for each autistic child should be a process akin to tailoring, in which different approaches need to be tried on. There may be a basic pattern and a logical sequence in which the first priorities have to do with cleaning up the diet and the digestive tract. However, each child should be viewed from a perspective that values individual differences, and does not simply seek to find ways in which the child resembles the other kids who share the autism label.

That being said, there are two ways in which we are all the same. One has to with the temporal domain of timing, rhythm, and tuning. The other has to do with the universally positive effects of plant protein, as compared with animal protein and the general rule that growing children will thrive on an intake of no *more than one gram per kilogram (0.5 gram per pound) of body weight. That's a rule for healthy children. Because our kids are not healthy, we need to monitor carefully the growth curves of children under treatment to make sure that their theoretical needs are being met. However, forcing large amounts of protein is usually not the answer.*

* * * *

For seven and a half years I tried to pile stones up to the heavens without having any base for my structure. Thus, nothing worked. With SCD securely in place, treatments that previously got me nowhere now move us up another inch or two closer to the cure.

The hardest part about writing this book is that I don't have an ending. I can't tell you that Alex is cured and we are all living happily ever after. Alex is not cured. Alex is still extremely sick and he's still profoundly autistic. But for the first time in a decade, we have some sort of quality of life. For the first time since he was born, I get to sleep more than three or four hours a night. He doesn't scream hour after hour anymore. He doesn't hit himself against the furniture and floor. He doesn't bite, scratch and mutilate himself to get his mind off the worse pain within.

For those of you reading this book and thinking, "My child doesn't exhibit self-injury! My child doesn't have any real gastrointestinal problems! My child sleeps fine!"—please, remember my story: "Every intervention we tried either did nothing or made Alex get worse." If your child's digestion is not working perfectly, he or she will not make the progress that is possible. It's that simple.

A few months ago, my boys were off from school for a week's vacation. One day we had nothing to do so I said to them, "Let's go bowling." And we did. The three of us went bowling. For those of you with children with autism, can you understand how wonderful this was? We went out to lunch together and then went bowling!

And Alex got a spare.

CHAPTER II

Irony, Bitterness and the Hippocratic Oath

*I swear by Apollo Physician and Asclepius and Hygieia and Pana-
ceia and all the gods and goddesses, making them my witnesses, that
I will fulfill according to my ability and judgment this oath and this
covenant:*

*To hold him who has taught me this art as equal to my parents and
to live my life in partnership with him, and if he is in need of money
to give him a share of mine, and to regard his offspring as equal to my
brothers in male lineage and to teach them this art - if they desire to
learn it - without fee and covenant; to give a share of precepts and oral
instruction and all the other learning to my sons and to the sons of him
who has instructed me and to pupils who have signed the covenant and
have taken an oath according to the medical law, but no one else.*

***I will apply dietetic measures for the benefit of the sick accord-
ing to my ability and judgment;*** *I will keep them from harm and
injustice.*

*I will neither give a deadly drug to anybody who asked for it, nor
will I make a suggestion to this effect. Similarly I will not give to a
woman an abortive remedy. In purity and holiness I will guard my life
and my art.*

*I will not use the knife, not even on sufferers from stone, but will
withdraw in favor of such men as are engaged in this work.*

Whatever houses I may visit, I will come for the benefit of the sick, remaining free of all intentional injustice, of all mischief and in particular of sexual relations with both female and male persons, be they free or slaves.

What I may see or hear in the course of the treatment or even outside of the treatment in regard to the life of men, which on no account one must spread abroad, I will keep to myself, holding such things shameful to be spoken about.

If I fulfill this oath and do not violate it, may it be granted to me to enjoy life and art, being honored with fame among all men for all time to come; if I transgress it and swear falsely, may the opposite of all this be my lot.[6]

This is the *actual* Hippocratic Oath.

The oath that new doctors swear at their graduations from medical schools these days is just an oath made up by each medical school for its own graduates, loosely based upon the original oath.

I for one didn't know that until I recently looked it up. And I can tell you that when I read the actual Hippocratic oath I was in shock.

Here's an example of a modern version, this one actually approved by the American Medical Association:

You do solemnly swear, each by whatever he or she holds most sacred: That you will be loyal to the Profession of Medicine and just and generous to its members. That you will lead your lives and practice your art in uprightness and honor.

That into whatsoever house you shall enter, it shall be for the good of the sick to the utmost of your power, your holding yourselves far aloof from wrong, from corruption, from the tempting of others to vice.

That you will exercise your art solely for the cure of your patients, and will give no drug, perform no operation, for a criminal purpose, even if solicited, far less suggest it.

That whatsoever you shall see or hear of the lives of men or women which is not fitting to be spoken, you will keep inviolably secret.

These things do you swear. Let each bow the head in sign of acquiescence. And now, if you will be true to this, your oath, may prosperity and good repute be ever yours; the opposite, if you shall prove yourselves forsworn.[7]

I can understand new doctors not swearing in the name of the ancient gods. Granted, the original oath could certainly use a bit of updating.

But...

"I will apply dietetic measures for the benefit of the sick according to my ability and judgment." Why did that clause land on the cutting room floor?

While reading about the Oath online, I came to the Web site of the Association of American Medical Colleges and found an essay entitled "A Hippocratic Oath for our Time," which opens with the following:

> It invokes Greek gods. It promotes nutritional therapy as the first defense against illness. It forbids euthanasia, abortion, and surgical procedures. It invokes dishonor and shame if it is sworn to falsely.
>
> Today's medical students are probably surprised upon reading the original wording of what has come to be known as the solemn vow each new physician takes when entering the medical community—the Hippocratic Oath.[8]

As I said, it's not only today's medical students who are surprised. After all those years of unsuccessfully searching for something to make Alex feel better, and finally learning of SCD through mothers—then to learn that the first medical tenet of the real Hippocratic Oath commands doctors to use diet to treat the sick! It left me positively dumbstruck.

Before I launch into my attack on the current medical system, I will say this:

If I had to pick the one thing that makes me admire Sid Baker, it's the fact that he abides by the following: "In medical school I learned a lot of new words. When you think about it, medical training involves learning to see and name invisibly small things, such as molecules, or invisibly large patterns, such as diseases.... In the course of learning the language of medicine, we learn four words that should never be said out loud: 'oops' and 'I don't know.' Successful collaboration between doctor and parents, in navigating the complex landscape of chronic illness in children, comes from an ongoing, leisurely, intelligent conversation in which the words 'oops' and 'I don't know' are allowed."[9]

When Sid saw the improvement in Alex, he simply said to me, "I'm sorry. I didn't know." And I forgave him. Sid doesn't have all the answers and he knows he doesn't have all the answers. Like us mothers, he is always trying to find them and always willing to learn. Sid didn't have his patients on SCD. Now he does. In fact, he's put as many of them on SCD as he possibly can.

Algernon: The doctors found out that Bunbury could not live, that is what I mean—so Bunbury died.

Lady Bracknell: He seems to have had great confidence in the opinion of his physicians. I am glad, however, that he made up his mind at the last to some definite course of action, and acted under proper medical advice.

– From Oscar Wilde's The Importance of Being Earnest

---

* * * *

Dr. Baker: *I have a companion to Judy's quotation from Oscar Wilde. It comes from Evelyn Waugh's* Brideshead Revisited. *Lord Marchmain has returned to his estate and family with his mistress, after living for many years in Italy. Upon his arrival home, his mistress, referring to his terminal illness, says to his family:*

"...The doctors in Rome gave him less than a year. There is someone coming from London, I think tomorrow."

"What is it?"

"His heart. Some long word at the heart. He is dying of a long word."

Just below, Judy will refer to our slavery to the prescription pad, where medical tradition scribbles the names of remedies for words that the language of medicine makes us believe are not mere names for but the causes of our problems. Prescription-pad medicine depends on a mythology that sees diseases, not individuals, as the targets of treatment and the causes, not just the names, of illness.

* * * *

This is certainly not the place to launch into a diatribe on all of the problems inherent in our current medical establishment. It is, however, the perfect venue to rail against one of them, namely the all-too-prevalent scenario of the expert doctor, with paternalistic condescension, talking down to the thankful and worshipful patient. Of course, doctors have their medical expertise. They have learned their biochemistry, anatomy, physiology. However, it is the patients who are the best clinical observers of disease and the effects of treatment because they are living with it 24 hours a day. Especially in the case of complex chronic illness, it is absolutely vital that the doctor and patient work together as peers. It is equally vital that patients have extensive opportunities to talk to others in the same situations, not only for the emotional support, but because most of the time, at least in my experience, patients are the best source of new information.

This commentary by Sid makes me laugh out loud every time I read it, and states clearly the necessity of having patients talk to patients: "I have fallen into a medical practice where I get to see more rolling eyeballs than a stripper. You should have been a fly on the wall when I started telling people about the Specific Carbohydrate Diet. Parents who had developed an unreasonable confidence in my opinion were pulling on their earlobes and staring out the window waiting for me to stop telling them about yet another impossible diet. It would take forty minutes just to get people to say—after my best trapeze act—that they would read the book and think about it. Then I got parents who had already tried it to talk to the ones who were trying to run back from the end of the diving board. Time required: ten minutes."[10]

When Alex was first diagnosed—when, for the first time I became really involved with the medical profession—I too put an unrealistic reliance upon the expertise of the doctor. As I said earlier, I had my first conversation with another mother grudgingly, perhaps even disdainfully. I believed, like so many other Americans, in "modern-day medicine." We've all become slaves to the prescription pad. If there's a pill that can fix things, we're popping it. There is certainly blame on both sides for today's lazy person's medicine.

Truly, it's not until someone you love becomes gravely ill that you really understand the limitations of what physicians can do. I'm not blaming them for their ignorance. I fully understand that science can only progress at a given rate. However, I do blame the medical profession for its close-minded arrogance and its sell-out to the pharmaceutical industry.

Physicians make mistakes all the time. Yes, so do the rest of us. But then again, most of us do not have life-and-death decisions to make every day. **Therefore, there is no profession where it is as critical to identify and remediate mistakes.**

Here are some of my personal favorite examples of "oopses" in medicine, in just the past few years:

1. According to the Institute of Medicine, 44,000 people died of mistakes in hospitals in 1999.[11]

2. In August of 1998, the FDA approved a vaccine for Rotavirus (one possible cause of childhood diarrhea) and this vaccine became a part of the normal vaccine schedule starting in January of 1999. The virus is responsible for approximately 20 infant deaths a year in the United States.[12] About six months later, in July 1999, the CDC pulled the Rotavirus vaccine out of use, saying: "This action was based on the results of an expedited review of scientific data presented to the ACIP by CDC in cooperation with the FDA, NIH, and Public Health Service officials, along with Wyeth-Lederle. Data from the review indicated a strong association between Rotashield and intussusception (bowel obstruction) among some infants during the first 1-2 weeks following vaccination."[13]

3. According to the *Journal of the American Medical Association*, there are

- 12,000 deaths per year due to unnecessary surgery
- 7000 deaths per year due to medication errors in hospitals
- 20,000 deaths per year due to other errors in hospitals
- 80,000 deaths per year due to infections in hospitals
- 106,000 deaths per year due to negative effects of drugs

Thus, America's healthcare-system-induced deaths are the third leading cause of the death in the U.S., after heart disease and cancer.[14]

4. On the CDC's Web site:

Simian virus 40, or SV40, was discovered in 1960. It occurs naturally in some species of monkeys, though it does not typically cause symptoms or illness except in cases where the animal has chronic problems with its immune system (Shah and Nathanson, 1976).... Soon after its discovery in 1960, SV40 was identified in polio vaccine. It was found in the injected form of the vaccine (IPV), not the kind given by mouth (OPV). At that time, rhesus monkey kidney cells, which contain SV40 if the animal is infected, were used in preparing viral vaccines. Because SV40 was not discovered until 1960, no one was aware that polio vaccine made in the 1950s could be contaminated. In 1961, the virus was found to cause tumors in rodents (Eddy et al., 1961). That same year, the federal government required that new stocks of polio vaccine be free of SV40. However, existing polio vaccine stocks were not recalled and were used until 1963. When SV40 was discovered, researchers did not know if the virus could negatively affect people's health. Many viruses that harm animals have no effect on people because of the biological differences between animals and humans.

Interest in SV40 has increased in the last several years because the virus was found in certain forms of cancer in humans, for instance mesotheliomas (rare tumors located in the lungs), brain, and bone tumors (Carbone et al., 1994; Jasani et al., 2001). More recently, SV40 has also been found to be associated with some types of non-Hodgkin's lymphoma (Shivapurkar et al., 2002; Vilchez et al., 2002).[15]

In other words, in the 1950s and early 1960s, Americans were being inoculated against polio with a serum that was grown in monkeys and was contaminated with a monkey virus that is now causing various forms of cancer in humans. Please take note: even after the virus was discovered, "existing stockpiles were not recalled."

My point is this: The Specific Carbohydrate Diet (originally referred to as the banana diet) was created by Dr. Sidney Valentine Haas back in the 1940s. In 1951 he published his book, *Management of Celiac Disease*. It's not that Dr. Haas was unknown and his diet an obscure bit of medical esoterica. The fact is, he was a very well-known pediatrician and his work was well accepted, based upon more than 50 years of research by himself and many other physicians over the decades.

He received a full obituary in the *New York Times*, which reads: "In 1924 Dr. Haas reported to the scientific world his probably most important contribution to pediatrics, the banana diet in the treatment of celiac disease, in which the small child cannot tolerate most of the starchy foods that are vital to him. Before the curative effects of the banana were reported by Dr. Haas, one of four celiac patients died."[16]

Several years earlier, the *New York Times* reported on a major award given to Dr. Haas by the New York Academy of Medicine, whose officials stated: "On his ninetieth birthday and his sixtieth year as a fellow, the New York Academy of Medicine extends its warm congratulations and good wishes to Dr. Sidney Valentine Haas and presents this citation with respect, affection and gratitude for his long years of devotion to the academy. As a scientist, he has contributed to our knowledge of the diseases of children. As a clinician and teacher, he has exemplified the highest ideals of the practice of medicine. A benefactor of children, he has, more than that, been a friend to man. In honoring him as a fellow, the academy does itself honor."[17]

So, whatever happened to the work of Dr. Sidney Valentine Haas? I do not know. His banana diet was a well-respected, extremely successful treatment for various intestinal diseases. Yet, over 50 years after his book was published, his work has essentially been completely forgotten, ignored, dismissed or purposely erased from the knowledge base of the current medical profession.

The only person who continued to carry his torch, for many years entirely on her own, was Elaine Gottschall.

Elaine: brilliant, funny, fiery, and most of all tenacious. However, Elaine was "just a mom," and therefore (unfortunately for tens of thousands of suffering people) was not one to gain the attentive ear of the collective medical profession. She had a master's degree, but not an M.D. or a PhD. Worse still, her message, should it reach even some of the receptive ears of individuals suffering from celiac disease, traditional inflammatory bowel diseases (Crohn's disease and ulcerative colitis), or autistic enterocolitis, would cost the pharmaceutical companies millions upon millions of dollars in unsold medications. Perhaps it is cynical of me (I am not a cynic by nature, but I am sure you will forgive me this one moment of weakness), but the way I see it, Elaine never did have much of a chance of winning this battle.

For more than 40 years, Elaine did everything possible to restore the Specific Carbohydrate Diet to its previous status as a standard medical treatment. She devoted her life to bringing what is often a cure for horrible intestinal disease back into the forefront of medicine. In the end, not surprisingly, it has not been the doctors who listened to her, but the patients themselves.

Elaine Gottschall came upon the Specific Carbohydrate Diet when looking for a way to save the life of her own young daughter, who was severely affected with ulcerative colitis. When a relatively simple dietary change completely reversed this supposedly incurable illness, she devoted herself to first educating herself in biology and nutrition, then researching the diet, then writing *Breaking the Vicious Cycle* to tell the world what she knew, and finally to helping families, one by one, to start the diet and have the courage and stamina to stick with it. When I was about to pull Alex off the diet after almost three months of no improvement, it was Elaine who reached out to help me—a complete stranger. She had seen my post on the SCD bulletin board *PecanBread* and wanted to give me the support to stay with it. Because of that phone call, for which I will be forever grateful, I did stay with SCD for that one more month....

On PecanBread's bulletin board: November 24, 2003, 4:45 PM:

> *Hi all. I am a new member of this group although I have been reading the postings for several months now (since I first started the diet with my son). Alex is 9, quite profoundly autistic, and has been sick most of his life—severe digestive problems and immune suppression. I've done everything out there—this is my last hope.*
>
> *Within 48 hours of starting the diet, Alex developed very severe diarrhea which lasted two weeks. We then had about 6 weeks of slightly improving behavior (less stimmy, less hyperactive, better eye contact, improved appetite), but the diarrhea continued on and off.*
>
> *Two weeks ago Alex had a huge regression. Now, I know that this is not uncommon, but it was quite severe and is still going on. I know that I shouldn't despair but... he's not eating at all, he's lost 4 pounds in a month (and he's already underweight), the diarrhea continues unabated... and all of the improvements we'd seen have vanished.*
>
> *I need to get calories into him. Does anyone have any ideas? Or even just stories like this where you found the light at the end of the tunnel. I don't want to give up yet...*
>
> *Judy*

November 24, 2003, 4:54 PM (posted in reply, nine minutes after mine):

> *Judy,*
> *Please call me Tuesday morning about 9:00 a.m. EST 905-349-3443.*
> *Elaine*

I don't think there's much question among those of us whose life she has touched: Elaine Gottschall is a true modern-day hero.

It's not much wonder that I have something of an attitude problem. Alex was on five or six medications at once to try to get his colitis under control. Even with those, he still suffered in screaming agony. All that time, all I had to do was remove complex carbohydrates from his diet. All those years of suffering... that's all I had to do.

* * * *

Dr. Baker: *Carbohydrates represent one of three main classes of food substances. As the name suggests, carbohydrates are molecules that consist of carbon and water (hydrate, as in dehydration, means water—from the Greek hydor). Carbohydrate molecules come in forms and sizes that differ in the way they are digested and absorbed when we eat them. Glucose—also known as dextrose—is simple sugar that is the same as the sugar that circulates in our blood. Like fructose, which is found naturally in fruit, it is "simple" in the sense that it represents the smallest unit (monosaccharide) of sugary molecule.*

When eaten, these simple sugars pass directly into the bloodstream without need for prior disassembly (digestion). When combined in pairs (disaccharides), small groups (polysaccharides), and long chains (starches and celluloses), they must be reduced (digested) to their simple components before they can pass from the digestive tract into the bloodstream to be stored or used for energy or as raw materials for making other molecules.

(Fats, another class of food substances, are also made of carbon and water but their atoms are arranged in ways that make them insoluble in water. As such, they have a very different path into the body. They still require digestion, but once rendered into simple units, those units pass into the bloodstream by first entering lymph ducts which do not pass to the liver but convey dietary fat via a pencil-thin tube in the back of the chest to be dumped directly into a big vein beneath the left collar bone. Sounds weird, doesn't it? But that's the anatomy. The third major classification of food is protein, which is distinguished by containing—along with water and carbon—nitrogen, which is 80% of the air we breathe but only becomes captured in useful form by bacteria working in conjunction with the roots of certain plants, such a legumes.)

The distinction between simple and complex carbohydrates is not very sharp on a chemical level, but for practical purposes, simple carbohydrates taste sweet and complex carbohydrates do not. There is a big distinction, however, between the main single-unit carbohydrates—glucose and fructose—and the disaccharides—sucrose and lactose. Sucrose is a double unit, combining glucose and fructose; lactose (the sugar found in milk) combines glucose and galactose. (The latter is a monosaccharide found in sugar beets and some plant gums and made by mammals out of glucose for the production of lactose in milk.)

When I first heard the term "Specific Carbohydrate Diet" I thought, "That's odd, what's specific as regards carbohydrates?" I confess that I never asked Elaine where she or Dr. Haas got the notion of "specific." It sort of turned me off to the idea and, like many doctors, I was blinded by a word that stuck in my ear rather than being open to digging beneath the semantic surface to understand the real issue. The real issue in SCD is, of course, the distinction between the innocent cellulose and monosaccharides on the one hand, and the guilty disaccharides, polysaccharides and starches on the other. That distinction isn't so much about the complexity of the carbohydrates as it is about their digestibility. We don't digest cellulose at all—it is the fiber that passes through us or is digested by our flora quite downstream in the gut to produce substances like butyrate that nourish the cells that line our colon. We don't need to digest monosaccharides—they pass directly into the blood as I just explained. The whole point of the SCD is that it addresses the problem some people have digesting the double sugars sucrose and lactose and other disaccharides (maltose, cellobiose) formed during the digestion of starches. **This is the specific point of SCD—that these disaccharides are strongly bound together and therefore hard to digest.** One of the first weaknesses to show up in the digestive tract if something goes wrong—from a passing infection or poor nutrition—is a weakness in the digestion of double sugars. A vicious cycle begins when these undigested sugars pass into the habitats of germs that normally inhabit the intestine. The germs can digest these sugars. When germs digest sugars, that's called fermentation. Even the cleanest fermentation for making wine or beer produces alcohol, which has certain toxic properties. Fermentation in your gut is not clean and produces mischievous gasses and other poisons. The additional damage to digestion of starches that results (hence the vicious cycle) is one of several kinds of mischief caused by these products of fermentation.

> ...each bit of goodness
>
> that each of us does
>
> to help others grows
>
> and grows and grows.
>
> – Elaine Gottschall

* * * *

For 40 years Elaine was a maternally enraged David, throwing one small stone after another at the medical Goliath. She was one woman against the colossus. But each one of these stones rose up to become a mother, and one by one, the numbers of her army grew.

The day I started Alex on SCD, I got a phone call from a friend with a daughter on the spectrum. "Judy," she said, "I was just online looking at things that help with Crohn's disease. I found this diet called the Specific Carbohydrate Diet and I've just read that it seems to be helping kids with autism." Speechless with shock for a moment, I stared down at my desk, which had *Breaking the Vicious Cycle* sitting on it (as I had just put it down to pick up the telephone). "Kate," I said, "I was just sitting here reading the book."

Sometimes it's hard to believe that coincidences really are just coincidences.

My friend and I helped each other through those first really hard months on SCD. When Alex started to show some improvements, I told my friend Stacey about the diet. She joined us, putting her four-year-old son on the diet. Then we were joined by Jessica, and then by Stephanie, Brenda, Heather, Sharie, two more Stephanies, Mona, Candace... Finally, our email inboxes were so full that I started a private bulletin board for us. Still our numbers continue to grow.

> *We don't care what they all think.*
>
> – My Dad, Wallace Chinitz, Ph.D.

There's no force like a bunch of parents who are dedicated to finding a way to help their children.

I tried to discover how it was that SCD first came to the autism world. Me, I'm a relative latecomer. Alex has been on the diet for more than three years but obviously, since I'd heard of it several years before that from a mom of a child with autism, there was someone out there way before me. Who was it who paved the way for us?

"Who was the first mom to try SCD on her autistic child?" I asked Elaine. "I don't know for sure," she told me, "But you should certainly talk to Mimi. Mimi had to be one of the first."

So, I talked to Mimi.

Mimi is another mom. She has a son on the spectrum, and two more children who have benefited from SCD for a variety of complaints. Mimi has been actively trying to spread the SCD message in the autism world for about six years now, ever since she first heard of it back in 1999. How did she hear of it? She tells me that there was an Internet chat room for adults with inflammatory bowel disease, the Long Island SCD listserve, and the group included *one* mother who was using SCD to cure her ASD child. Also, there was another mother, the owner of another bulletin board called Recovered Kids, who was an SCD proponent. I checked Recovered Kids. The first post was December 2, 1999. So somehow, somewhere, it occurred to a mother that what worked for those with recognized bowel disease might well work for her child with the new diagnosis of autistic enterocolitis.

I thank them all from the bottom of my heart.

For years I'd suspected that Alex was affected by something akin to traditional inflammatory bowel disease. After all, in 1998, I heard Andrew Wakefield describe autistic enterocolitis as "a subtle variation on Crohn's Disease." In November of 2002, when Alex finally had his colonoscopy, I had that suspicion confirmed. However, it never occurred to me to research how people with these related disorders were treating themselves. In retrospect, I can't understand what I was thinking—or more accurately, not thinking. The wisdom of hindsight is pretty painful sometimes, but not as painful as the thought, "What would have happened to Alex if it weren't for these other mothers?"

One by one. Inch by inch. Elaine says, in her introduction to Raman Prasad's book on his experience with SCD and ulcerative colitis, "We have a saying among us Specific Carbohydrate Dieters which reads, 'we will reach one person at a time and will keep planting seeds.'"[18]

CHAPTER III
Elaine Gottschall

he·ro (hîr´ō)
*A person noted for feats of courage or nobility of purpose,
especially one who has risked or sacrificed his or her life.*

– Dictionary.com

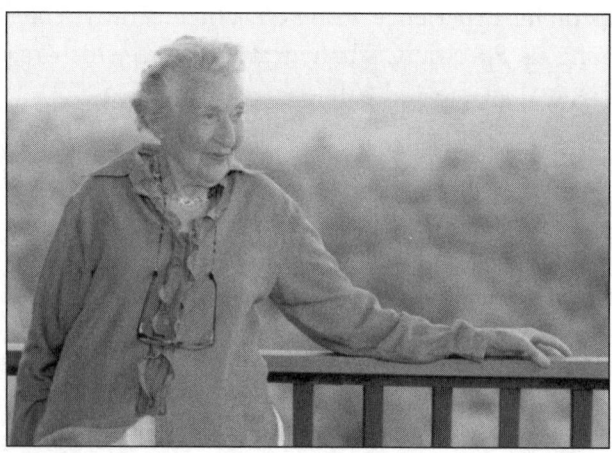

Elaine was a remarkable woman. Truly remarkable. A force of nature.
The first time I spoke to her on the phone, the call that gave me the cour-

age to keep Alex on SCD, I hung up thinking, "That woman has more energy than everyone I know, combined." Subsequently, I found out that she was 82 years old.

It never actually occurred to me that anything could ever happen to Elaine. When you were with her, you never thought about her age. She was just Elaine, full of passion, fun, laughter, and joy. One evening, at the DAN! conference in Boston, in April 2005, Elaine and I sat drinking in the hotel bar. We talked about everything from the state of Alex's liver to the state of Western medicine. We talked about ourselves and the coincidences that to us made a pattern of our lives. Her daughter, whose illness introduced Elaine to the Specific Carbohydrate Diet, thereby setting the course of her life, is named Judy. Elaine and her husband were married on my birthday. She met him at my alma mater, Columbia University. I said to her that she needed to write her autobiography: her life was such a remarkable testament to the power of the individual that she needed to have it down in black and white for all to read. She agreed to work with me on a book and a couple of months later she began to write her notes for it.

From Elaine:

I was born in a suburb of Pittsburgh, Pa. on August 18, 1921, at home. My Mother had carried two pregnancies before me to completion but the children died a few days after birth.

So, I was welcomed and loved to high heaven but by a very sick mother who had had kidney problems and was told after the second pregnancy not to have any more children. But there I was!

She adored me and I think that first year of love gave me the strength to carry on through the rest of my life—up until Judy became ill.

I was an active child and was into everything. My German granny called me in German "a mixing spoon"—Koch leffel.

We were poor so the small house was filled with a large family of adults. One was my wonderful grandmother (Mother's mother) who rocked me and cared for me during the many times when my mom was too sick to do so. Then there were three sisters of my mother's, and two brothers (one was to become the doctor, Uncle Phil, and one supported the rest of the family by having a large newsstand at the busiest corner of downtown Pittsburgh).

When I was disobedient, all I heard was, "You are bad, no one will love you and your Mother has been sick from the day you were born." I would say, even at the age of two, "I will love myself if no one loves me," and I thought, "Oh, how I want to be good!" But most of all I KNEW that I did not make my mother sick and I think that was the start of my losing respect for authority figures and what they proclaimed. If that is the start of believing in yourself, then it started there!

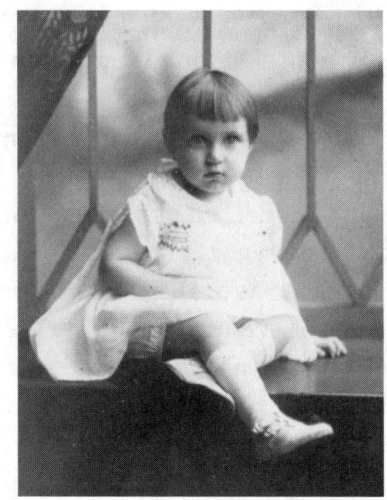

But, many years later, when a gastroenterologist at NY Cornell told me I was to blame for Judy's colitis, I would die before I believed this and thus began the fight of my life to save her and save me.

When I learned that Bettelheim was blaming mothers for their autistic children (way back in the 1950s), although I did not have an autistic child, I developed a kinship with those mothers. Little did I know that I would be thrown in with them some day. I recoil when I detect any hype that throws blame back at the victim.

During the time of my mother's illness, I developed a social conscience about the practice of medicine. I felt that "it's not bad enough that one falls victim to disease, but then the doctors take all your money from you and still don't deliver." (Years later, as a high school student, I wrote my English term paper on different types of medical systems, and when the opportunity came to move to a country with a social net for medical care, I chose to move to Canada.)

Because my father did not succeed in business, and because it was during the Depression years, I was forced to move every school term. Each September, up until junior high, I was in a new school. From Pittsburgh, to Brooklyn, back to Pittsburgh, to Baltimore, back to Pittsburgh, and on and on. When we finally did settle down in 1936 in Baltimore, I put roots down for the first time and did very well in school. But half a year before I was to graduate with my class from Forest Park High in Baltimore, my Mom died and I was forced to move in with relatives in Brooklyn.

I remember writing back to my class at graduation time:

I think about you all so much
And yet I can't explain
It's like a hopeless case, that freezes up my brain.
I want to see you march that night
before you say goodbye
I want to see that flag point upwards to the sky
But most of all I want to say
How lucky you are friends
To know that Forest Park and you
Were pals until the end.

I have never gotten over not graduating with my high school class.

I started Erasmus High School in the last half of my senior year, had to make up for all of the regent exams that I had not taken and I got my diploma. All dreams of going to college were smashed. I went to secretarial school for three months and got a job in 1940 for $15 a week in Rockefeller Plaza.

The war was on. I continued working as a secretary and sold war bonds in front of the Astor Hotel every night. How I remember the mobs of people at Times Square. At the start of 1943, after a few trips back to Pittsburgh and my father's death, I returned to New York and decided to change jobs. Little did I know that the employment agency across the hall from the ladies' washroom at my old job was recruiting office help for the Manhattan Project. When they sent me to Teacher's College at Columbia for an interview, I thought I would be working for some faculty member. I passed my dictation test but was told the job they had for me had just been filled. (Later I learned they had to do an FBI check on me before hiring me.) In two days, they called again and this time gave me a map of the campus and told me to go down three flights of stairs after entering Schermerhorn, the geology building. When I descended, I saw two guards standing at a barricade and when I gave them the pass, they opened the door to the "beginning of my life."

The first person I bumped into was introduced to me thus: "Elaine, this is Herb Gottschall and he won't forget your name because his fian-

cée's name is Elaine."

I thought, "Oh, what a lucky girl!"

He was one of the golden boys who had just graduated from Yale; the others were all Ivy Leaguers from engineering, chemistry, and physics with a few Nobel Prize-winning professors running to and fro. One night as I sat minding my own business and typing, I heard a voice say, "How about some dinner?" Here was that gorgeous Herb asking me out—but he was engaged. We went to the deli on Broadway near 128th and sat there for three hours with the chemistry working like mad. The next morning, I asked his friend about his engagement and was told Herb had broken it a few months prior to this.

The next months were magic. We had New York to ourselves. We had dinner at Tony's on West 53rd almost every night and walked hand-in-hand back to Central Park West where I was living with my aunt. On my birthday, August 18, 1944, there was a small package on my typewriter with my engagement ring. We were married on October 8, 1944.

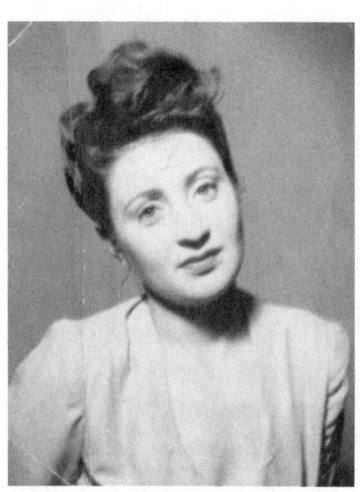 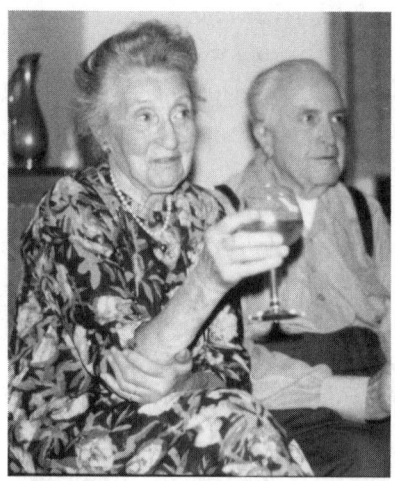

[Herbert Gottschall died on December 22, 2000, of Alzheimer's disease. In a separate email, Elaine wrote to me of his death:

"Herb had started developing Alzheimer's about eight years before he died. I watched him slowly go and swore I would never send him to an institution. In the meantime, I was a wreck every day. The kids

said I needed a psychologist so I went and he told me to institutionalize Herb and I refused.

But on December 1, 2000, I could no longer cope and we put him in a nearby facility and he died three weeks later. He knew me and he didn't know me. It is so maddening—all our memories—all gone most of the time. But the last words I said to him when I left on the night of the 22nd were 'who am I?' He shook his head and I said 'I'm Mother Goose and who are you?' And he answered 'Mister Goose.'

He was smart until the end."]

The pilot plant project at Columbia University (separating U235 from U238) was completed and we had a choice of going to Los Alamos; Pullman, WA; Chicago; or Oak Ridge, TN. Because Herb's parents lived in Jackson Heights, in Queens, we chose the eastern location of Oak Ridge so they could visit us easily. Joan was born in Oak Ridge on April 23, 1947, and we could have remained at Oak Ridge or chosen to leave. So leave we did, with our five-week-old baby and went back to New York. There was little in the way of housing, so we moved in with Herb's parents with whom I had a good relationship. However, as soon as we could we found an apartment in New Jersey where Herb had a job (Rutherford) and Judy was born there.

Judy was born on December 23, 1952. She was full-term but I was in labor almost 48 hours when the obstetrician couldn't get a strong heartbeat and had to go in with forceps. The cord had almost choked her and he pulled her out very quickly, according to the nurse (he left for Bermuda immediately after delivery). Unlike Joan, who had been chubby and pink and beautiful, she was blue from the forceps and her straggly black hair was all over the place. In spite of all that, I nursed her and within a short time, she filled out and was a beautiful baby.

However, even for a nursing baby, her bowel movements were very watery and very frequent. She also seemed to have night sweats as she was wet with perspiration when I lifted her out of her crib in the a.m.

The diarrhea persisted for months, during which time the pediatrician had me scrape apple and give her Kaopectate, neither of which did a damn thing. I remember that I did try to take an evening off and leave her with a sitter but I was so nervous I spent most of the time in the washroom throwing up.

I felt that my milk was doing her no good although her weight seemed normal, so I weaned her at four months. I don't remember what formula I gave her but things went from bad to worse. At about eight months, she had period of severe constipation intermittently with the diarrhea. Then, when she was around one year old, she began having nosebleeds. These increased in frequency for a long time, occurring sometimes during sleep and often as we were having a playtime—just suddenly and for no apparent reason. Sometimes I could pack her nose and stop the bleeding; sometimes we had to go to the ER.

At about three years of age, she began having the seizures—a very special kind. They occurred one hour after she fell asleep. The first time it happened, Herb and I were watching TV and we heard this ear-piercing shriek. We ran in to find her standing up in her bed, perspiration dripping down her face, her eyes wide open. She screamed in terror. She lashed out with her hands and screamed that we were killing her and we had to restrain her to keep her from flinging herself down the steps or onto the floor. We tried smelling salts and brought her beloved dog up to her room, but nothing fazed her. She saw nothing—she was in another world!

These episodes happened about three or four times a week. Our doctor said, "All children dream." I knew this was different even from the type of thing that occurs with high fevers. Shortly after the seizures started, about three months later, she awakened at 2 a.m. and rushed to the bathroom. This was the first time she did this. She sat on the toilet until 7 a.m. and I couldn't get her to get off. Finally, I led her back to bed and went to flush the toilet—and it was filled with blood.

We rushed down to our family doctor and he turned white. (I didn't know he had recently buried a young nephew who had died of ulcerative colitis.) We called my uncle (an internist in Pittsburgh) from the doctor's office and he gave me the names of the top pediatric gastroenterologists in New York City. Oh, God!—what an animal the first man was! He hospitalized her and wouldn't let us visit. He gave us the diagnosis of ulcerative colitis and put her on cortisone, and we had to follow up with potassium supplements. I remember how horrendous those supplements were. Three times a day, I would try to get a teaspoon into her of this foul-tasting stuff into her and she would proceed to vomit everything up.

But the bleeding stopped, the diarrhea stopped and she gained back weight.

I was so naive, I thought she was cured. Sure, she grew hair in her pubic area and under her arms, and sure, she turned into a tomboy, which she never was, and sure, she lost hair from her head by the handful—but the bleeding and diarrhea stopped.

When the doctor weaned her off, the symptoms returned in about two months—and this time the prednisone did not work. He told us she would need the colectomy.

Herb and I went crazy. We started the parade of doctors. We went to Leahy in Philadelphia, we went to the Mayo Clinic, we went to about eight other GI men, but they said the same thing: "food has nothing to do with it." (My common sense told me otherwise.) They insisted that surgery was the only answer for our four-year-old. My uncle and I were on the phone constantly. He said to bring her to Pittsburgh and I did. He started her on sulfasalazine (Azulfidine) and watched her for a week at his home. We came home and it seemed to help a little. But the symptoms were still there, although a bit milder. We had to do bimonthly blood tests, etc., and we had some chilling experiences with false results of the tests. By the end of one year, we started on the doctor hunt again. It looked like she was going to die... so back we went to the New York Cornell Medical Center.

When we started making arrangements for the surgery, I began to cry. At this point, this doctor said, "What are you crying about, Mrs. Gottschall? You've done this to her!" I went home with her and went into my bedroom, closed the door and cried for about two days nonstop.

This is one of the most distressing stories I can imagine, and what happened to Elaine also happened to many moms of autistic kids in years past. Doctors blamed them outright for their children's condition: the legacy of the highly influential developmental psychologist, Bruno Bettelheim. Until 1964, when Dr. Bernard Rimland wrote Infantile Autism—which told the world that autism was a physiological condition—it was thought, thanks to Dr. Bettelheim, to be the fault of "refrigerator mothers" (unloving, cold mothers who rejected their infants).

It was then that a friend called and came to visit. On her way to see me, she stopped in the supermarket and bumped into a third person and told her about Judy. This woman said, "Tell your friend to call me immediately and I will give her the name of the doctor who saved our celiac twins." I called and she gave me Dr. Haas's telephone number and within 48 hours we were at 91st and Park Avenue with all the blood test reports and stool culture reports that we had collected within the last year.

* * * *

Dr. Baker: *Medical misbehavior, like every other kind of misbehavior, has roots in laziness, greed, pride, lust, anger, and envy. I believe, however, that the main cause of really stupid medical behavior is shame. When doctors feel ashamed that they don't have the answers they tend to lash out at patients.*

The simplest stupid medical blame-dodge can be set up in the following way: The doctor establishes a strict regimen of diet or medication. You follow it. You return and you are not any better. The doctor finds that there was some imperfection in the way you adhered to the directions. Now it is your fault that you have not improved. You are a bad patient. Actually, Mother Nature is more forgiving than that and will generally permit healing if you get it mostly right.

Elaine, Judy, and many other people have been victims of a more complex shame-and-blame game. Here's why it happens. We doctors are engaged in a high-stakes effort (the stakes being your health) that demands thinking about the worst-case scenario on the one hand and hoping for the best-case outcome on the other. We are vulnerable to being ashamed when we don't have the answers. That shame is a powerful force that makes us wish to cast blame elsewhere.

Now consider the possibility that many of the diseases we confront in the population we serve are iatrogenic—that is, caused by the medical profession. Not in the sense of an individual physician's negligence or bad luck, but in the collective sense of complicity with, or acceptance of, the possible dangers of common medical practices. We protect ourselves with consensus. As you may know, when I graduated from medical school in 1964, the firm medical consensus was that autism was caused by "cold mothering." In retrospect, this was utter nonsense and without any basis in reality, as Dr. Rimland's book Infantile Autism *articulated so clearly and effectively.*

Nowadays we have other points of consensus. Antibiotics pose little risk to the individual—even though it is a fact that they always cause a disturbance of the intestinal flora, and the intestinal flora have proven, metabolic, endocrine, immune, and toxicological functions that are very important. Immunizations are generally so safe that they are exempt from the same policies that ensure a modicum of safety from pharmaceuticals—*even though multiple immunizations are often given in one visit, and many contain toxic materials. There is a sense that if we are all doing it, we are protected by the consensus. There is beneath the surface, I believe, a haunting sense that these collective beliefs and practices—along with a general disregard of nutrition—may not withstand scrutiny, and thus we don't want to take a peek at the reality. Instead, we stupidly blame patients for problems that we cannot solve and so, as individual physicians, manifest a sort of collective sense of shame for our failure to stand guard.*

I find my patients' families reluctant, especially upon first meeting me, to tell tales about things doctors have said to them about the causes of, and outlook for, their children's problems. Such tales as Elaine and Judy report are common. If you have experienced such abuse, you should tell the tale because telling your story is one of the most important factors in healing the injury caused by having a physician cast blame upon you.

* * * *

That was as far as Elaine got. She sent me the last installment on May 5, 2005. She then went away to speak at a conference for a few days and when she got back, she sent me an email:

> *Judy, I am too nervous with this circulation problem in my leg to concentrate right now so I will try to get back to our story when I know more about what is causing it.*
> *Love, Elaine*

On May 28, sick with worry after not hearing from my friend for several days, I called and emailed. In response, I got this email:

> *Judy, I have sat here for an hour wondering if I should tell you this. But I will eventually have to, so here goes.*
> *My leg swelled up awfully today so I went to the ER. They did a CT scan and I have a tumor in my pelvic area which is pressing on a blood vessel. So early next week, I should have it removed.*

I am numb about it all and hope it all turns out all right.
Much love.

Elaine Gottschall died of cancer three months later, on September 5, 2005.

Her family gave me the great honor of writing a eulogy, which was read at her funeral. I had only a few minutes, so I couldn't express everything I wanted to say. I am including it here because I want you, my readers, to have it:

While I can't be with you all today, I am very grateful for the op-portunity to have a few of my words read. Elaine was my friend and my hero. She called me her adopted daughter. I love her more than I can say.

We met two years ago because, with her seemingly infinite com-passion, she reached out to help me when I was at the lowest point in my life. My son, Alex, who is profoundly autistic, was then nine-and-a-half. His colitis and cryptitis were so severe that he was starving to death. I was a complete stranger but Elaine read of my troubles and found the time to talk to me. She kept me going.

I think that the best tribute I can give her is to tell you what her work meant for just my one little family. We're a microcosmic example of how much suffering in the world one person can alleviate by just giving a damn. When I met Elaine, Alex was horrifically self-abusive as well as completely destructive. His way of asking me for help was to rip our house to shreds, as well as his own skin and body. I couldn't even take him to the supermarket, between his destructive behaviors and his continual and unending need for a toilet.

On the day Elaine passed away, not knowing that she'd had a downturn over the two previous weeks, I sent her this email. It says everything I need to say: thank you, Elaine, for saving my son, me, and our family, and for giving me the incredible blessing of your friendship and love.

Emailed on September 5, 2005:
Dear Elaine,
I hope you're feeling better and recovering as rapidly as possible. I was hoping to find an email from you when I got home from Europe

two days ago... I haven't heard anything on your condition since before I left. If you're feeling well enough, please just email me even one line to tell me how you are. I miss you very much.

I hope this helps you to heal: Elaine, I just flew to England and back on my own with the boys. In the midst of that we flew to Greece for a week. Your friend, Alex, was INCREDIBLE. Calm, smiling, happy—he couldn't have been better behaved on the airplane journeys. In fact, the flight attendants didn't even realize there was anything wrong with him. He was sitting quietly, eating snacks, watching his little DVD player... and they kept coming up to him to ask him if he wanted water or juice, etc. He was an angel.

My friend Tracy, who hadn't seen him in two years, was literally crying when he went up to her and said, "Play catch." They played catch in the park for at least 15 minutes, with Alex smiling, laughing, and making eye contact with her the whole time.

So I'm sending some of our healing right back at you. In my life, I never thought I'd be able to comfortably take Alex to the supermarket, let alone on a two-week trip to Europe. We went to restaurants (the Greeks were amazing about cooking his food specially), sightseeing, boating, swimming... just like normal people.

I know you've gotten a million of these emails from me, let alone from other people over the years, but this one is special. It comes with more gratitude and love than you can fathom.

Much love,

Judy

I am so thankful that I had two years of Elaine. And I am so thankful that I have this book. When I write, it brings me close to my friend. It lets me carry on her battle in my own way.

Elaine can't finish her autobiography herself, but as far as I'm concerned, she and I are still writing this book together.

"We are winning, Judy. Maybe you and I should write a book together... We have a lot of people on our side now."

In her notes about her life, she had just gotten up to the climactic moment: the moment she met Dr. Sidney Valentine Haas. That was the moment that changed her life and, through her, my life and Alex's life. Trying to continue to use Elaine's own words as much as possible, I will fill in that blank using this transcription from her speech at the DAN! conference, October 2004, in Washington, D.C.

> *Good morning. It's been a long, long journey. And I'm not talking about the flight from Toronto, Canada, to Washington, D.C. Before I give you a few highlights of this forty-year odyssey I've been on, I want to express my appreciation to all of you; but a few people stand out. Dr. Rimland, thank you for taking the albatross of guilt from these courageous parents and for relentlessly pursuing the causes… and eventually we will find the cure for autism spectrum disorders….*
>
> *It was 1960 when I had a defining moment in my life. I was sitting in the pediatric gastroenterologist's office of New York Cornell Medical Center with my seven-and-a-half-year-old daughter and we were being prepped for surgery to have her colon removed. She had been diagnosed with very severe ulcerative colitis three years before and the medications had ceased to work and he was going to make the arrangements for the surgery…*
>
> *We had gone in a period of two or three years to 12 or 15 gastroenterologists and they said that if the medications didn't help, surgery was imminent. And now I was sitting in this office and being told that, yes, we will schedule her for surgery. I began crying and this doctor pointed his finger at me and said, "What are you crying about? You've done this to her." Yes, I know all about Bettelheim.*
>
> *At any rate, I went home and closed my bedroom door and cried and cried and couldn't stop. And then, something interesting happened. A friend called and said, "May I come and just talk to you, Elaine?" "Oh sure, Martha." And on her way up she bumped into a third person and told her about me, and this woman said, "You have your friend call me and I will give her the name of a doctor in New York City who saved our two celiac twins, saved their lives." And I jumped out of bed when Martha told me and got Dr. Sidney Valentine Haas on the telephone. And within 48 hours, carrying my latest pathology reports in one hand and stool culture reports in the other hand, we entered his office. And after a thorough examination, he sat me down and he said those very famous words, "Mrs. Gottschall, what are you feeding this child?" None of the twelve doctors—not only did they give me no information on diet, but when I asked about it they said that it had nothing to do with*

intestinal problems. In fact, even today, were you to go to a gastroenterologist—most of them, not the ones here!—and ask them, for your Crohn's Disease or your colitis, what to eat, they would say, "Doesn't make any difference. Food has nothing to do with it."

He sat me down and I said, "Dr. Haas, she's really not eating very much and what she does eat goes right through her or she throws it up." He said, "OK, we're going to change all that." I want to tell you people who are struggling about whether to start SCD because you're afraid of it, this was a piece of cake. In 20 minutes, Dr. Haas gave me one, two, three. Nothing written down, not even the yogurt recipe. He said, number one, you've got to get her off all fluid milk. But because milk has so many good nutrients in it, protein and calcium, we will make our own yogurt. We'll ferment it 24 hours. You can make milkshakes with it. She can have natural cheeses. They have no lactose in them. He was concerned with carbohydrates. That was nothing. I could do that. Number two, she cannot have any table sugar or anything that has table sugar in it. That includes maple syrup, a very natural product, but unfortunately it has sucrose in it. She cannot have corn syrup, but she can have honey. Don't believe it when they tell you there's no difference between honey and sugar. The molecular structure is different.

He told me that for years, sick children and babies were given honey because it requires no input from an injured intestinal surface and it gives them energy: it gives them good, palatable food.

But the third thing he told me was a humdinger. She cannot have any potatoes or grains. I went home, and in the car on the way home

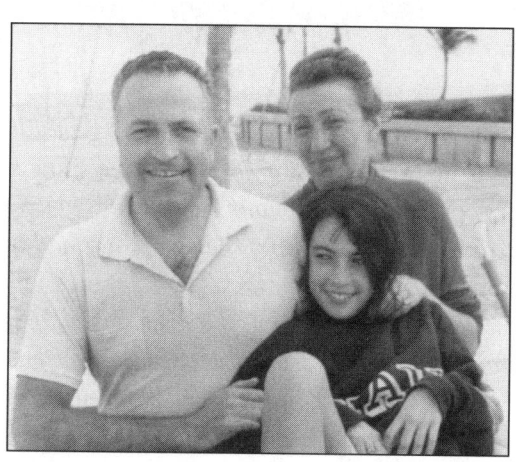

I thought, "How am I going to bake for this child? How can I bake her birthday cakes and cookies?" I had an Austrian friend who made beautiful nut tortes and I called her up immediately. She said, "Put some pecans in the blender and grind them up, put some eggs in, put some honey in, and you'll have great muffins."

I did that. I put Judy on the diet immediately. Within three days the night seizures went, never to return. My daughter is 51 years old now and has two beautiful children. That same gastroenterologist had advised me that she'd never have children. We have two beautiful, thank God, grandchildren and she's never had a return of the neurological symptoms. The colitis, we were out of the woods by the end of a year. And I caught my breath.

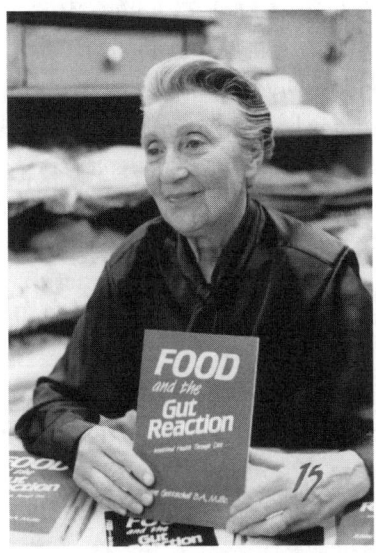

I had no formal university education. I had graduated from high school in '39 during the Depression. But I started going to the Rutgers medical library and within a half hour I found on the current periodical stacks evidence of some of the things that Dr. Haas had told me about. For example, milk intolerance, the lactose intolerance, had been known since before the 1900s and not one of these doctors had mentioned it to me. We had no Xerox machines. I copied the information down quickly and brought it home to my very positive husband, who heard me say, "I am so angry. We should have known about this. It had been published

from before 1900 and nobody told me." And then he said the famous words: "Elaine, you've always wanted to go to the university. There's one 20 minutes away, Montclair State." He said, "Get in there and find out what in the blankety-blank is going on around here. I have to make a living." So, like a good wife in the '60s, I took off... and I spent 12 years there. [Elaine went back to school to get her bachelor's degree at 48 years of age. She began work on her master's degree at 52.] *And when I turned 60 I thought, well, I'd had enough. I was halfway through a Ph.D. And I began teaching, doing consulting, and had garnered enough information to write my book.*

My search in the university had one goal and that was to go on a treasure hunt and to find out how something as simple as a diet could reverse an incurable disease. That was my 12-year treasure hunt.

Elaine devoted 12 years of her life to researching why it was that removing certain foods from her daughter's diet resulted in a complete cure. She then went on to write her book, *Breaking the Vicious Cycle*, the book that saved our lives. Her book has a copyright date of August 1994—Alex was almost six months old at that time. As much as I try not to, I have these thoughts too often: what if his pediatrician had told me about it when he was first diagnosed? What if that gastroenterologist at Mt. Sinai Hospital hadn't laughed at me but instead had told me to put Alex on the Specific Carbohydrate Diet?

But these "what if" thoughts get me nowhere. I try not to dwell on them.

Besides, Elaine wouldn't have wanted me to sit here thinking about my defeats of the past. Elaine was all for fighting on. Our conversations and emails were constantly infused with both her sense of hope and her conviction that it is up to the moms to lead the way. Elaine was entirely "willing to march into hell for a heavenly cause." So that you can all get to know her a little better, I will share her with you through those emails...

> *Compassion is not helpless pity, but an awareness and determination that demands action.*
>
> – The Dalai Lama

On receiving the official invitation to speak at her first DAN! conference:

Darling Judy,

Yes, I just received Dr. Baker's kind invitation.

I just could not give up—it has been a long journey and, so far, I am blessed with strength and conviction to keep moving.

I will reply to his invitation tomorrow. I am still digesting it. Just goes to show you that 'you don't fool around with us Moms!'

Much love

Judy, I may not have told you how much admiration I have had over the years for Dr. Rimland... In my introductory psych course in 1969, having just seen Dr. Rimland's landmark book on autism, I did my final psych thesis on his book. I have observed the autism community at almost every move. Bettelheim spoke at my university and a more contemptuous individual would be hard to find... But today is another beginning, I hope. I just keep telling myself to keep going because "we are not talking about chopped liver!"

...I am afraid that I will burst out in tears when I meet Bernie. He will never know how his work has impacted me. The whole idea of taking blame (by Bettelheim) off these desperate parents' shoulders is a very strong underpinning in what makes me "run." Scapegoating by ignoramuses of all stripes and colors! We Moms and Dads, so in love, so devoted to our children, working so hard to do the right thing—not only are all our dreams shattered but we are bearing the albatross around our necks. Our lives are practically destroyed... I know I will cry and he will think I am crazy.

Dear, dear Judy,

...I am so happy. Don't know why I was given this torch to carry but carry it I did and each day is more rewarding than the one before.

As I said earlier, Elaine always seemed filled with a joyous passion. Oh, she certainly got very angry sometimes. But she never seemed to dwell on the negative. Instead, her energy seemed to spring from the happiness she got when yet another person got better, another child stopped screaming.

"Dr. Moms are strong and feisty... and we will fight to our last breaths. Onward Soldiers!!!"

The worst of times for me, when I think I can't fight another day, are when I am flooded with the memories of all my failures for Alex. Sometimes I can't help but remember all the time I wasted not having him on SCD. One day I wrote to Elaine, telling her about a horribly painful experience I'd just had. I'd brought Alex in to our regular pediatrician for his annual school physical. "How's it going on SCD?" he asked me. "Great," I said, "Although I'm a little disappointed that so far I haven't seen much in the way of cognitive or language development." "Well, he said, "He is 10. And you know, when these kids get past that critical age..."

Of course, I've never gone back to that practice. "Past that critical age"... People in comas wake up after 20 years and no one knows how or why. People lose chunks of their brain to strokes and accidents, yet manage to recover fully, with parts of the brain taking over the functions of others. But this pediatrician knew exactly when I should have thrown in the towel. Amazing that with medical knowledge like that, he still hasn't managed to cure autism.

* * * *

Dr. Baker: *This is one of the most common myths of child development. It goes in the category of the magnification of small truths, which I referred to previously as a downside of the Internet's access to information (and gossip).*

It is, of course, a fundamental observation about human development that it is a sequential process in which windows open—and close—at various times and stages. Experiments in animals show how critical the timing is of certain healthful or noxious stimuli to the ultimate fitness of the adult creature.

Children's capacity for healing certain kinds of wounds decreases with age. For example, if a the tip of a child's finger—including the bone and nail—is accidentally amputated by, say, a car door, it was once the practice to attempt re-attachment or to suture the wound and accept the reality of the amputation. In a busy emergency room a child was once bandaged to await further treatment. Delay and misunderstanding led the parents to take the child home. When the family returned for a follow-up visit the doctors discovered that the fingertip had regrown—bone, nail, and all—thus revealing the young child's capacity to handle such problems if left to do so. Regrowth of the fingertips occurs before age five and not afterward. This kind of age cutoff, however, is not so clearly applicable to predictions about the developmental capacity of children in or near the autism spectrum. Many of our kids have potential that is buried in the chaos of a disturbed chemistry of inflammation, detoxification, and oxidative stress. If we support these children and allow them to heal, we will unearth treasures of language and creativity. The best outcomes come from early intervention; but do not accept verdicts rendered by professionals who make predictions based on chronological age.

* * * *

I don't usually succumb to idiocy, but the doctor's comment managed to pierce my armor. I was just devastated. I just love Elaine's response. It did cheer me up. She was good at cheering me up.

As far as [these doctors go], they know nothing, NOTHING about health—only stuff in bottles! Judy was eight years old, having schizoid seizures and falling into a serious neurological condition, until SCD. She snapped out of it. I am fully aware of how much we desperate parents need a line to a professional when hit by this stuff but, really, many of these people are wimps. Little boys/girls, educated in a certain way, made to think they are knights on white chargers out there ready to keep all of us from dying. But they know nothing about health!… Remember, Judy, they told me that our child would never have children!!! They are usually wrong. There is a cliché for medical students: "Half of what we teach you will probably be found out not to be true, but we don't know which half!"

One thing that did manage to upset Elaine was once again being confronted by a doctor whose refusal to listen was resulting in the continual suffering of a patient. One day she called in tears. Elaine in tears! The living version of the rock of Gibraltar was tired and worn out. We talked on the phone for a long time, commiserating. I wrote her an email that night saying, yes, sometimes it seems impossible to go on, and this was her response:

Judy, I'm supposed to be 'mothering' you and I had to wait for your email to be "mothered." It reminds me of Herb having to keep after me to keep going. How many times did I say (while studying those 12 years), "I have to quit. I can't stand it!" And he would say, as you just did with your email, "You know you aren't going to quit!" So, thank you, again, Judy darling.

I wish I had Elaine here to convey a better sense, with details, of the years she spent, after researching and writing her book, being quite literally laughed at by the medical community. For example, I specifically remember her telling me about a conference in the UK at which she'd been asked to speak. She was jeered at by some doctors during her talk. It was a very painful memory for her but it wasn't going to daunt her. She knew that SCD would help so many children with autism, and she kept her eyes on the prize:

> My own uncle, with whom I grew up, was only ten years older than me and I adored him. When Judy was going to be operated on, he told me to get on a plane and bring her down to Pittsburgh. He put her on Azulfidine (prednisone had been the only drug the bastard at NY Cornell had used and when it didn't work—the knife!) and it gave us another year. But a few years later, after she was well, I was in Pittsburgh at his home while his wife was getting dinner on the table, and he asked me about the "diet that cured Judy." I no sooner said one sentence with the word "carbohydrate" in it and his eyes glazed over and I lost him. They don't have a clue how to think other than drugs and surgery. And, remember, he liked me—almost like a younger sister—and he couldn't or wouldn't get it.

> Judy, what to do to help move SCD right along!

> Sid [Baker] did the most and if he continues to support us, other things will open up. As a result of DAN in D.C. and my talk in Toronto, at least six medical doctors are turning their practices over to using SCD… I do think the SCD wave is on its way. There are at least a few dozen doctors who are ordering the books in quantity in the USA. And these patients are being helped immensely. This word of mouth thing is powerful but slow…

> Without Sid, I could have gone on—one person at a time—and would have been satisfied. Better people than I have tried to change the world and have met with rejection and being treated like pariahs. Jonas Salk, in his book, The Green Years (written about 30 years ago) devoted about 25% of the book to talking about his problems with the Polio Foundation. Linus Pauling was constantly being ridiculed… Sid is as smart as they come; he found a way to do good without hurting the practice of his colleagues. He can't do all the fighting for us but—he opened the door for autism.

Elaine, when I am filled with despair, when I'm tired, when I feel like I can't bear Alex's illness or the suffering of my friends' children, I look at the photo of us together that sits on my desk and I think about your joy when you found out you were to speak at a DAN! conference. You knew how many more parents you could then reach and how much more suffering you could help alleviate. I think of this email all the time and I can't read it without feeling a little burst of an internal fire that says, "I'll *never* give up."

> *Oh, Judy, this is too much! I just can't believe this is happening. I think I died and am in heaven. We never know what it is like when we cross the gap. Maybe if we go to heaven, our lives continue the way we dreamed they might continue. I was thinking of this today. Everywhere I looked, it was sheer beauty—the countryside, my home, everything!*

> *Judy, I love you! The angels, the angels! They are around us, I know. And I don't want to make you cry again, but my Herbert Angel is here with me all the time—things come out of my mouth—decisions that I know can only come from him. I am glad you are "one tough bitch" because we are fighting a real war against every possible money interest out there. Not that I don't like a lovely standard of living, I do. But when it is a toss-up between their bottom line and the happiness and health of my loved ones, there is no hesitation as to how hard I will fight. You will be here to carry on when I am finally resting.*

Yes, Elaine, I am here. And I promise you that I will work as hard as I can to help as many people as I can. I am very lucky: I knew you. I knew Bernie Rimland. I had the best teachers in the world.

CHAPTER IV

The Specific Carbohydrate Diet

All truth passes through three stages. First, it is ridiculed. Second, it is violently opposed. Third, it is accepted as being self-evident.

– Arthur Schopenhauer

Over and over, parents tell me that while they are very interested in putting their children on SCD, they need help in learning how to organize themselves, how to get their children to accept new foods and giving up old ones, and so forth. I have spent many hours—more than I can count—on the phone talking parents through the fundamentals. Therefore, I thought it would be an excellent idea if I attempted to put down on paper what one of these conversations typically encompasses. I hope that here I can answer all those questions so by the time you're finished reading this book you'll be convinced not only that the diet is a necessity, but also that it is doable.

Think of this chapter as a reference guide. For ease of use, I have broken it into the following sections:

1. What is the Specific Carbohydrate Diet anyway?
2. Removing all your doubts, fears and excuses

1. What is the Specific Carbohydrate Diet, anyway?

Bad bacterial microbes—yeasts and unhealthy bacteria—produce toxins irritating to the lining of the digestive system, which cause the tissue to try to protect itself by secreting mucus. This is the normal physiological reaction to irritation. (Think, for example, about your runny nose when you sniff some pepper.) When covered by a thick layer of mucus, the intestines are unable to break down complex carbohydrates because the necessary enzymes (secreted by the intestines) can't reach the food, leaving the undigested carbohydrates (sugars that cannot be broken down into digestible form) to fester and feed the bad bacteria. All that great food lets the bacteria and yeast have lots of babies, as Elaine liked to say... which leads to more toxins... which leads to more irritation... which leads to more mucus... which leads to worse digestion....

Elaine's vicious cycle.

To quote directly from *Breaking the Vicious Cycle*:

"In various conditions, a poorly functioning intestine can be easily overwhelmed by the ingestion of carbohydrates which require numerous digestive processes. The result is an environment that supports overgrowth of intestinal yeast and bacteria... The purpose of the Specific Carbohydrate Diet is to deprive the microbial world of the intestine of the food it needs to overpopulate. By using a diet which contains predominantly 'predigested' carbohydrates, the individual with an intestinal problem can be maximally nourished without over-stimulation of the intestinal microbial population."

When you keep all complex carbs out of the digestive system, the aberrant bacteria are starved to death. Of course, at the same time, you're replenishing the gut with good flora. These good flora are also known as probiotics, and are ingested via the SCD-legal homemade yogurt and/or store-bought probiotics (which are available from a host of retailers).

SCD stops the vicious cycle of malabsorption and microbial overgrowth by removing the microbes' food: sugars, specifically di- and polysaccharides. Single-molecule sugars, like those found in fruit, vegetables, and honey, do not require digestive processes and are immediately absorbed by the intestine. Therefore, even damaged intestines can absorb them and they are not available to feed the bad flora. Inflammation decreases as the bad microbe population dies out.

To learn more about the many years of science behind SCD, I strongly suggest you read Elaine's book, *Breaking the Vicious Cycle (BTVC)*. It is available via Amazon.com, LucysKitchenShop.com, and BarnesAndNoble.com. *BTVC* is an easy read, in spite of the fact that Elaine goes into some detail on the scientific theory behind why SCD works. For the skeptics among you, there *is* a lot of science behind the SCD, but certainly not enough. It's not easy to get the dollars necessary to fund research into a diet. In a recent article in *Take Charge*, a publication of the Crohn's and Colitis Foundation of America, a Mayo Clinic doctor is quoted as saying, "Studies are expensive and someone has to pay... Most clinical studies in this country are funded by pharmaceutical companies... and since there's no potential drug at stake with this diet, it would be difficult to find industry funding." So, much is known about why and how SCD works, but much more research is needed.

However, it absolutely does work. Sometimes it works miracles. Someday, in the not-too-distant future, I hope that finally it will be accepted for what it is: **a fundamental treatment for bowel disease**.

Science does not yet have all the laboratory answers about SCD, but we do have plenty of clinical data. By now, I am assuming I have managed to convince you that it is absolutely imperative that you improve and modify your child's diet. Remember: the diet works almost all the time and even if it doesn't help, it can't hurt. It's simply the healthiest possible eating and good nutrition.

* * * *

Dr. Baker: *I agree with Judy that SCD is harmless in the usual sense of that word. Unlike a drug or an operation, it is not associated with sudden, serious,* unexpected dangers. On the other hand, any dietary change that eliminates certain foods will require you to make substitutions that may be problematic—especially as you go through the sometimes dramatic ups and downs that can occur in the initial and even later stages of the diet.

How can you know if negative symptoms are part of the adjustment to SCD or the result of an intolerance to foods that have been introduced or increased with the exclusion of sugars and starches? Here are some things to watch for:

First, weight loss. If children lose weight or adults lose more than a reasonable amount of weight or continue to do so after SCD has otherwise stabilized, then modifications are called for to determine whether the cause is insufficient caloric intake or malabsorption due to the effects of something new.

Another problem that sometimes arises with SCD is that it tends to result in a high protein intake. Just as a diet consisting of only sugar and french fries is not good for anyone, a diet consisting of health-food-store gluten- and casein-free hot dogs and homemade organic chicken nuggets is not good for anyone. We all have learned about dietary "balance" and about the "food pyramid" from authoritative sources who advise a healthy distribution of fats, carbohydrates, and protein. We have learned that protein is one of those three major food types required in good quality and good quantity—especially by growing children. We know that plant protein is "incomplete" and animal protein is "high-quality." All of that stuff is wrong. This is not a matter of changing dietary fads or shifting expert advice—which are enough to make most of us take refuge in some general notion of "just eat a balanced diet." It is a matter of a very new understanding about the relationship between diet and chronic illness.

The understanding is not all that new; it has been around—published at the highest level of science, for a few years. But I, who have thought that I knew quite a bit about nutrition, was blind to that understanding until April 2006, when I was invited to give a lecture about detoxification at a national meeting. Speaking at the same meeting[19] were scientists from teams of researchers who have been looking at the fundamental factors underlying the kinds of chronic illnesses that are prevalent in affluent societies such as North America: heart disease, cancer, allergic and autoimmune disease, dementia, attention deficits, mood disturbances, autism, and so on. I cover the topic more extensively in the 2007 update of Autism: Effective Biomedical Treatments. Moreover, there are two books that will fill you in on the whole story: The China Study, by Colin Campbell, and Eat to Live, by Joel Fuhrman. I urge you to read these two books, which you will find enormously reassuring as to what you can do to prevent and/or treat most of the chronic health problems that we worry about these days.

I would like to tell you the basic take-home messages here because they have a strong bearing on SCD. First, animal protein is not more "complete" than plant protein taken from a variety of sources, such as cereal grains, nuts, and beans. Second, in the context of the environment in affluent industrialized societies, consumption of animal protein has serious negative effects. Among meat, fish, eggs, and dairy sources of animal protein, the casein found in milk products is the most dangerous. Finally, we should eat organic fruits and vegetables not just because organic food is richer in vitamins and minerals (which is true), but because organic fruits and vegetables are richer in phytonutrients. What do I mean by phytonutrients? Substances that plants make to protect themselves. They are, in effect, often the toxins that plants make to minimize their attack by pests—bacteria, fungi, insects, and other animals. These toxins comprise a long list of substances whose names we are beginning to see in popular nutrition literature. They are—again, in the context of modern industrial societies— more important in some ways than the vitamins and minerals and essential fatty acids and amino acids that have been so much the center of nutrition science in my lifetime.

Why? Because they address the central factor in the diagram I presented before, that shows the three overlapping circles of the chemistry of autism. They are the same three circles that form the underlying features of the biochemistry of all the chronic illness I just mentioned. We have been taught that different diseases all have different causes, but that turns out to be a misleading perception. It is more true to the facts of life that in any ecological setting the common (prevalent) problems tend to be linked to common (shared) factors.

At the center of the diagram is GSH, which is reduced glutathione, the biochemistry of which links detoxification, inflammation, and oxidative stress. The phytonutrients I mention have diverse actions, but their nearly universal function has to do with the induction of GSH. Induction. That's a key concept that underlies the way this group of nutrients plays a role in the prevention of cancer, heart disease, etc. You know the adage that if you give a man a fish he can have supper that night but if you teach him to fish he can eat every night? Well, induction of GSH is a much better way of approaching the problem of low GSH levels in our kids than is giving GSH. Not that giving GSH is bad. Not that we shouldn't take measures to improve thiol chemistry with elimination of heavy metals and other toxins and supplying methylcobalamin to help convert a vicious cycle back to a virtuous cycle of thiol chemistry. But now that we know that substances found in broccoli sprouts, for example, have a powerful capacity to induce GSH, we have access to tools that have not caught our attention in all the complexity of dietary intervention for children in the autism spectrum (and those with other problems that share autism's underlying chemistry).

So let's come back to the question of how to avoid the possible negative effects of SCD that may come from over-consumption of animal protein and how to maximize the beneficial effects of phytonutrients that induce GSH. First, be aware that growing children need about 1 gram of protein per kilogram (about ½ gram per pound) of body weight to sustain growth. The point is that more than that should be viewed as more likely to be bad than good. What if digestion and absorption are problems, as they are in many of our kids? More reason to be careful about excesses of the indigestible food. The idea is to fix the digestive problem—break the vicious cycle that has to do with abnormal flora—and not simply to pour in more of the troublesome foods, which now include both starches AND animal protein. Second, if SCD provokes negative responses that indicate a problem with phenolics, salicylates, or oxalates that are found in fruits, nuts, and/or vegetables, be aware that the very foods that you may pull from your child's diet to avoid these "toxins" carry phytonutrients that are essential to his or her health.

I know that I am raising crazy-making issues. Those of us who are trying to sort out the biochemistry, immunology, and toxicology of autism have traveled many tedious miles through the dietary swamps that tax the intellect and patience and imagination of the most skilled parents, who already have a lot of other things to deal with. To simplify things, here are some basic rules to steer by:

1. Minimize the amount of animal protein in your SCD to the extent possible.

2. Minimize the length of time you wait in hope that the vicious cycle referred to in Elaine Gottschall's book will be broken. We could never get a simple answer from Elaine on the question of how long it takes. Of course, every person is different. Before I learned about the problems associated with animal protein, my general feeling was: when in doubt just keep the SCD in place. For a while I thought that it might be how everyone, including me, should eat. Now I think that unless you can do a plant-based SCD without weight loss or keep animal protein to an absolute minimum, SCD should be treated as a temporary measure to last only long enough to break the cycle.

3. *If you run into complications that indicate problems with some components of fruits, nuts, and vegetables, whose consumption is increased with SCD, be careful to test—by repeated avoidance and challenge—to see which specific components or specific fruits, nuts, or vegetables are the culprits. Try not to simply get a list of all foods containing oxalates, phenolics, or salicylates or colorful components and stop them because those are the very types of foods that provide the benefits our kids need the most.*

4. *Be aware that some negative reactions to fruits, nuts, beans, or vegetables (as well as gluten and casein) are allergic and as such may be specific to a particular food as opposed to a whole group of foods that happen to contain, say, salicylates. Testing for allergy to a suspected specific food is pretty simple. Take it out for five days and then challenge for three days. Repeat the process until you have enough clues—anything from behavior or digestive symptoms to minor indicators like red ears or stuffy nose—to make or break the case.*

5. *Keep your sense of humor and don't be a prisoner of dogmas about what is or isn't bad for "autistic kids." Remember that Mother Nature has a sense of humor that she expresses by being inconsistent about a lot of the things we are discussing. Thus, your child may react differently to a food on different days. Fanatical strictness has its place in this dietary minefield, but try to avoid taxing yourself with exacting expectations without knowing the penalties for leniency.*

* * * *

2. Removing all your doubts, fears and excuses

My background is in special education. I was originally licensed in teaching the blind and visually impaired, but when Alex got sick, I refocused myself to learn more about general special education, specifically ABA, and I got recertified. I am not an ABA fanatic. I see a lot of flaws in the way it is too often practiced, but that's another story. However, I most certainly am a behaviorist at heart. It is through the general principals of behavior modification—appropriate and desired behaviors are rewarded—that I managed to teach Alex to actually eat real food.

When he was diagnosed at two years of age, like many children with autism, he ate nothing except bread, crackers, Cheerios, and pretzels. A fruit or vegetable touching his mouth inevitably resulted in vomiting. The occasional chicken nugget would be the sum total of his protein intake. He ate only crunchy foods, never anything soft. He wouldn't even drink from a regular cup. At the very sight of anything but his sippy cup he would throw himself onto the floor and scream like he was being murdered. To say that Alex had severe tactile defensiveness is a vast understatement.

Now, at almost 13 years of age, Alex eats meat, fish, fruit, and vegetables (he particularly loves sautéed mushrooms, onions, and zucchini), drinks from a cup, uses a fork and spoon...

So, how did I do it?

Perseverance. A willingness to put in the effort now for the payoff later.

That's it. That's the whole secret.

I want to take a moment to review with you the message behind one of the best-known of all fairy tales. Without consciously realizing it at the time, we've all been taught a valuable lesson starting early in our childhoods.

"That's not the way to build a house!" he said. "It takes time, patience and hard work to build a house that is strong enough to stand up to wind, rain, and snow, and most of all, protect us from the wolf!"

The days went by, and the wisest little pig's house took shape, brick by brick. From time to time, his brothers visited him, saying with a chuckle:

"Why are you working so hard? Why don't you come and play?"

But the stubborn bricklayer pig just said no.

"I shall finish my house first. It must be solid and sturdy. And then I'll come and play!" he said. "I shall not be foolish like you! For he who laughs last, laughs longest!"

– from www.AllThingsFrugal.com

Put in the work now, build that house of bricks, or spend a lifetime regretting it. The fact is that you *can* change your child's eating habits, no matter how daunting it may seem. It is not impossible.

I won't lie to you: it may not be easy at first. But it is most certainly entirely doable, and you won't regret the effort you put in.

You'll only regret *not* putting in the effort later, when you look back and think, "If only..."

"If only..." The words that haunt me. If only someone had told me about SCD when Alex was first diagnosed.

Trust me: You don't ever want to have to say "if only."

I got Alex to eat new foods simply by being more stubborn than he was. He could—and did, in fact—spend years screaming, crying, trying to get out of first his high chair and then his regular chair, spitting out the food... and I'd just not give in. "You *will* learn to eat real food, Alex," he heard over and over. "Unfortunately for you, you got me for your mother. I'm more stubborn than you are! This is not a fight you are going to win." I'd pair a bite of something he didn't want with a bite of something he did. I used one-for-one reinforcement. Meal after meal, day after day, I'd sit with him, and as soon as a bite of chicken went into his mouth, or a bite of a vegetable, I'd quickly stuff into his mouth the piece of cookie or the chip he really wanted. (This was, of course, way before I'd ever heard of SCD. Back then, I used whatever gluten-free treats he wanted.) Now he eats a normal variety of foods.

So, yes, you may be in for a rough few months. Your child may have a complete, screaming meltdown when he or she finds out that the potato chips are gone, the days of ice cream and french fries are past. But if you persevere, you will have your child eating a wide variety of healthy foods.

3. SCD basics

Now that we've established why SCD works and why it is that you must do it—as well as demonstrating that it *is* possible to get your child to eat new and healthier foods—a discussion of how to actually implement SCD is in order.

First of all, you must understand what your child is permitted to eat and what is illegal on SCD.

To start with the latter category: any food that contains disaccharides and polysaccharides (that is, double and multiple chains of sugars) is illegal. These include table sugar (disaccharide) and any grain or starch (polysaccharides). Fluid milk is also not permitted on SCD, and non-aged cheeses, because these contain lactose, which is a disaccharide.

However, the good news is that the list of permitted foods is very extensive, and the even-better news is that there are legal substitutes for almost any well-loved favorite.

Here is a brief summary of what is permitted and not permitted:

LEGAL FOODS	ILLEGAL FOODS
Non-processed proteins, such as meat, fish, eggs, natural cheeses (must be aged), and homemade yogurt	Processed meats, like deli meats; breaded proteins, like fish sticks and chicken nuggets; coated meats, like honey ham; fluid milk or any type of dried milk products; commercial yogurt
Almost all vegetables are permitted (fresh or frozen)	Canned vegetables; **all** grains, including rice, wheat, spelt, corn; potatoes (both white and sweet); soybeans; starchy vegetables, like parsnips, chick peas, turnips
Almost all fruit (fresh, dried, or frozen) is permitted. Canned fruit is allowed as long as it is in its own juices with no added sugars. Bananas must be eaten only after they are fully ripe (that is, they have brown spots) because unripe bananas still contain starch.	All sugar (except fruit). (Be careful with canned tomato products: many contain sugar that may not be listed on the label. Use Knudson's tomato juice instead, or make fresh tomato sauce.)
Nuts	
Fruit juice, fresh or frozen. Be sure no sugar has been added.	Soy, rice, commercial almond milk
Oils of all sorts, including those made from corn and soy; butter	Margarine

No one expects you to memorize the list of every legal and illegal food. I have been doing SCD for more than two years and I certainly have to double-check things on occasion. I highly recommend you organize yourself by getting a three-ring binder to keep in your kitchen. Go to Elaine's Web site, www.BreakingTheViciousCycle.info, and click on the "legal/illegal" list. Print the entire thing and put it in the first section of your binder so that you have it for easy reference. Other things I keep in the binder include recipes that I get off the Internet or from friends, as well as instructions on making yogurt and anything else that I may need to refer to quickly.

One other important note: Doing this diet involves more cooking than most of us are used to doing. There's just no way to get around it. Few packaged foods are legal, and to make sure your child isn't accidentally ingesting illegals, it's a good idea to make everything from scratch. That's the bad news. The good news is that recipes tend to be very simple and not particularly time-consuming, and also, almost everything freezes beautifully. Cook in bulk and freeze. It will make your life much easier.

Now that you understand what foods are permitted on SCD, your next step will be to decide how you want to start the diet—cold-turkey, or gradually. Your decision will be based upon many factors. Here are some things to think about:

A. Have you ever had your child tested for food allergies? If not, you may want to do this before starting SCD. Many children on the spectrum, because of their faulty immune systems and leaky guts, have many food sensitivities and sometimes severe and potentially deadly allergies. When food substances leak through damaged gut walls, they cause the body to react as if it were being invaded by enemies. Undigested food should never end up in the body. The digestive tract is meant to be a closed system. The immune system will react to the invaders with an inflammatory response: that is, allergy. As SCD allows the walls of the gut to heal, less and less undigested food will be able to pass through the intestine; subsequently, the aberrant inflammatory response will decrease and sensitivities will fade away. However, true allergies, like a nut allergy (as opposed to nut sensitivities), will tend to be enduring.

* * * *

Dr. Baker: *Your digestive tract comprises a surface area about the size of a tennis court. How can this be when the tube we are talking about is, at most, about 22 feet long and a few inches in circumference, with an apparent surface area more like the size of your kitchen table? It has to do with its texture, or surface architecture. If you inspect your tongue closely you will see that it is not smooth; rather, its surface is composed of a crowd of velvety projections. Up close, the surface of velvet is not defined by its apparent dimensions but by the trip a microscopic traveler would make from the base to the tip of every single strand of fiber the makes up the nap of the velvet's surface. Farther down your digestive tract in the small intestine, the surface consists of a double-velvet of which each strand of the surface pile is itself velvety so that the collective surface* area is multiplied enormously and provides space for a lot of business to be done in a hurry. That business has to do with a selective permeability allowing for the absorption of nutrients—mostly small molecules that are the products of digestion—and the exclusion of big molecules that still carry the complexity of their origin.

That is, you are not supposed to get "eggy" from eating eggs in the same way you get garlicky from eating garlic. As it happens, a small amount of egg, wheat, milk, or other proteins and germs in our food does get absorbed into the bloodstream where it is "tasted" and remembered and later recognized by our immune system. The immune system's job is completed when such foreign visitors are cleaned up in a process that requires sticky labels (antibodies) being applied to the visitors which are then gobbled up by cells that read the labels. The selective absorption of good things and exclusion of bad things fails when the velvet of the digestive system is damaged. The damage may be the cause or the outcome of toxic, allergic, and infectious events. For example, allergy to a food such as egg may result in a "rash" on the intestinal surface, just as poison ivy or a certain cosmetic may cause a rash on your skin. Once damaged in this way, your intestine loses some of its protective capacity to exclude unwanted substances. It becomes leaky—in the sense of a tendency for excess substances to pass from the digestive tract into the bloodstream.

The idea of a leaky gut, as this situation has become known professionally and popularly, has captured our imagination since lab tests were introduced in the 1980s to measure the appearance in the urine of test materials (special kinds of sugars) that should pass unchanged with or without being absorbed from the intestines into the bloodstream after being swallowed. Because the test requires a timed urine collection, it is not easy to perform in little children. Because gut inflammation is nearly universal in children on the autism spectrum, a leaky gut is assumed to be present and to be the mechanism associated with many clinical and biochemical features, including food sensitivities and the trouble done by food molecules that look like our own mood-altering messenger molecules (opioids). Keep in mind, however, that a leaky gut is just one of many phenomena that may be causes and/or effects as participants in the many vicious cycles that get going in chronic illness. Thus, avoiding an allergenic food, such as egg, yeast, milk, or citrus, may help heal a leaky gut—or treating an infection may, by fixing a leaky gut, help get rid of a food allergy.

* * * *

There are two types of serum (blood) allergy testing: IgG and IgE. Simply put, IgG tests for sensitivities over a long period of time, as in constant exposure to commonly eaten foods that leak through the damaged gut wall. IgE testing, on the other hand, identifies substances capable of causing an immediate and severe allergic response. For example, an IgE allergy to nuts means no nuts, ever.

Because the baked products in SCD are mostly made with nuts, it is a good idea to make sure your child doesn't have an IgE reaction to these foods (which include peanuts, even though peanuts are technically legumes). Of course, if your child has been eating nuts all along, this is unnecessary. For most of our kids, however—especially those whose typical diet consists of french fries and pretzels—nuts are a new addition.

It is also good to have an idea of IgG food sensitivities and avoid these foods for a while, until the gut has time to heal. By avoiding them, you will lessen your child's inflammation and speed healing.

Foods that have shown to cause a reaction should be introduced slowly and only one at a time, after several months of avoidance. This way you can know for sure whether your child is actually reacting or not.

If you are unsure about your child's food allergy situation, discuss with your doctor the idea of running IgG and IgE testing before starting SCD so you will optimize the chance that the new foods you introduce will be well tolerated.

I was able to start SCD with no lead-in time with Alex because he was already nine and a half years old and had been tested multiple times for food allergies. Plus, I had already done allergy-avoidance diets with him multiple times before, and I knew that avoiding his "sensitive" foods made no difference in his health or behavior.

---

* * * *

Dr. Baker: *Allergy as a medical specialty had its beginnings 100 years ago. Its first decades coincided with a trend toward putting the practice of medicine on a more scientific—that is, measurable—footing. As a result of this trend, individuality took a back seat to categorization. This makes sense when one is* talking, say, about the predictable relationship between certain causes (such as germs) and certain diseases. However, allergy is by its very nature an individual affair.

Thus the specialty of allergy had a steep climb to medical respectability. It was helped along by the discovery of certain kinds of antibodies—eventually called IgE—that were associated with hives, asthma, eczema, hay fever, and other expressions of sensitivity to pollen, dust, mold, food, and chemicals. But science's demand for clear definitions and measurements was a tough terrain for the clinical realities of manifestations of allergy that did not fit neatly into boxes or could not be readily explained by scientific principles. The practice of skin testing to identify the cause of allergic symptoms involved methods that required a lot of art—as did various methods of desensitization that involved deliberate periodic exposure to small amounts of the offending substances. The impulse to be "scientific" took the practice of allergy more and more toward pharmaceuticals, as antihistamines and steroids became standard tools for suppressing the immune response.

As allergy/immunology achieved standing as a medical specialty, its scientific leanings triumphed over empiricism and practitioners established boundaries that excluded consideration of problems that were not "standard" inflammatory problems of the skin and respiratory tract, such as eczema, asthma, and hay fever. The central nervous system, delayed sensitivities, food allergy, and chemical intolerances were off-limits except to a group founded in the 1930s by clinicians whose modern legacy is the American Academy of Environmental Medicine. The notion that mood, hyperactivity, attention problems, and fatigue can stem from food allergy is still heresy among most allergist-immunologists. The idea that such symptoms can result from delayed or cyclic reactions to food or chemicals, or that they can be correlated with antibodies other than IgE, is also largely unaccepted by mainstream allergy practitioners and academics. Apart from semantic issues, the controversy boils down to this: to what extent do we wish to map nature to our neat map of reality largely based on lab tests—or, conversely, to accept the messiness of individuality while driving decisions in which the patient's response is the final word?

IgG is a family of antibodies. These constitute the repertoire of long-lasting antibodies that serve the memory we carry of every exposure we have had to every foreign substance from the time germs and dirt entered our bodies with our first breath and first food. They are, to a large extent, reflective of ongoing exposure, so that a blood test for IgG antibodies correlates with your diet. Such *a blood test can be useful if the results are taken with some grains of salt that are specified in my part of* Autism: Effective Biomedical Treatments. *The point is that IgG testing should not be used to eliminate foods from your diet beyond a trial period of a couple of weeks at the most to see if avoiding the reactive foods makes a difference. The larger point is that we should not restrict healthy foods, such as fruits and vegetables, without convincing evidence based on symptoms, not lab tests, that such avoidance is beneficial.*

* * * *

B. Does your child eat a wide variety of foods or is he a very picky eater?

If your child is already a good eater—a rare thing in the ASD population—then switching to SCD won't be a problem. The foods are delicious. If, however, your child is a chicken-nuggets-and-french-fries-only kid, it's a better idea to begin the diet slowly to avoid negative situations for both of you. As the parent of a child on the autism spectrum, your life is stressful enough. Fighting over every single bite of food at every meal for what could be weeks is not a good idea.

Start by substituting one food at a time. For example, if your child loves cookies, make some SCD-legal ones and replace the old favorites. If he objects, go back to my behavioral suggestions above: for every one bite of the new cookie, give a bite of the old. The next time, make it two bites of the new for every one of the old, and so forth.

Three or four days later, make your next substitution. Continue this pattern for the next month or two and before you know it, not only will your child be entirely SCD-legal, but you will have gotten rid of all the junk food in your house.

One of the most common questions I am asked is: what about chips? Almost all of our kids are chip-aholics. I use a couple of chip substitutes with Alex. Pork rinds are perfectly legal, if not the healthiest food in the world, so the occasional bowl of pork rinds is certainly fine and kids love them.

Another good substitute is dried apple chips. These are very crunchy, taste wonderful and are also readily available at stores like Trader Joe's (and online at various sites, including www.DigestiveWellness.com). I recently bought a dehydrator and plan on trying out other foods, like squash. The longer you dehydrate, the crispier foods get.

The second most common question I get about substitutions is: what do we do about french fries? Yes, this is a tough one. Sliced butternut squash, deep fried or baked in the oven with olive oil and salt, makes a very decent replacement. The truth is, though, that for the first couple of months, your child may well miss those trips to McDonald's. French fries were Alex's number-one favorite food before SCD. We would drive past those golden arches and invariably, a little voice would emanate from the back seat, "french fries." Alex remains barely verbal, but those were two words he never had trouble with. However, after a month without fries, he stopped asking for them and was perfectly content with other snacks and treats. As hard as it might be to believe now, your child will forget.

C. Are all the necessary foods readily available in your area, or will you need to order things via the Internet? If you live close to a good health food store, you will be able to buy nuts free of additives and can grind them into nut flours if you want to start SCD right away. However, the best nut flours (finely ground makes better baked goods) really are available via the Internet alone. Digestive Wellness (www.DigestiveWellness.com) has many available. Lucy's Kitchen Shop (www.LucysKitchenShop.com) has what I think is the best almond flour, at a very reasonable price. Also, Nuts4u (www.Nuts4u.com) has a wide variety of products available.

Don't start SCD until you are comfortable with the foods you have in the house, or you'll just end up frustrated. Good preparation will make the transition much easier.

Whether you decide to go cold turkey or to introduce the diet gradually, a great way to organize yourself is to write down a list of what your child is currently eating and then next to it write what an SCD-legal version will be. Here is what Alex's chart looked like when I started:

CURRENT FOODS	SCD-LEGAL VERSION
Breakfast	
Dry cereal	No cereal is allowed—no substitute
Gluten-free muffins	Muffins (made with almond or pecan flour)
Gluten-free waffles	Waffles (made with almond flour)

Lunch	
Peanut butter sandwich	Peanut butter sandwich (almond flour bread)
Chicken nuggets	Chicken nuggets (coated with almond or pecan flour)
Cheese sandwich	Cheese sandwich (made on almond flour bread with cheddar cheese)
Cookies	Cookies (made with almond, pecan, or other nut flours)
Fruit	Fruit
Dinner	
Pizza	Pizza (made with an almond flour crust, tomato sauce, and cheddar cheese)
Rice or potatoes	Stir-fried vegetables or squash
Hamburger	Hamburger, minus the bun, with veggies and cheese on top
Meat (lamb, steak, chicken, etc.)	Meat (lamb, steak, chicken, etc.)
Snacks	
Potato chips	Apple chips
Fruit	Fruit
Raisins	Raisins
Pretzels	Dried fruit

Mind you, this is a bit misleading because before SCD, Alex would often go for days without eating anything at all. So, the above chart was based on what he might eat on a good day. As you can see, there were substitutions available for almost everything Alex ate, so going onto SCD wasn't nearly as hard as I'd thought when I first picked up BTVC.

Also, you've noticed that I've included foods that contain casein. When I started Alex on SCD, he was still on a casein- and gluten-free diet. However, years of him getting nothing but sicker on this diet had demonstrated to me that casein was not a factor. (To test this theory, I had put casein back into his diet multiple times over the years with absolutely no difference to either his health or his behavior.) I started SCD exactly as Elaine Gottschall described it in her book, which means that cheese is legal. However, based on what I have learned since then, I would not recommend using casein immediately when starting SCD. (See my discussion of this later.)

4. Familiarizing yourself with the available resources

I believe it is absolutely crucial to read Elaine Gottschall's book if you're considering SCD. She provides an eloquent and easy-to-understand explanation of the history of the diet and the decades of science that support its efficacy, as well as providing some of the best SCD-legal recipes. *Breaking the Vicious Cycle* is available via Amazon.com and BarnesAndNoble.com, as well as through some of the SCD Web sites, which I'll list in a moment. It is *the* formative work on the diet and I for one consider it nothing less than monumental in its importance.

I have three SCD cookbooks and love them all. All three are available from LucysKitchenShop.com or from Amazon.com. They are:

1. *Lucy's Specific Carbohydrate Cookbook* by Lucy Rosset (has great basic recipes including my all-time favorite cookie recipe, her cinnamon raisin cookies).

2. *Adventures in the Family Kitchen* by Raman Prasad (has wonderful recipes of all types, including several amazing Indian recipes that my whole family—including extended, non-SCD family—loves).

3. *Grain-Free Gourmet* by Jodi Bager and Jenny Lass.

There are multiple Web sites devoted to SCD legal products, yogurt machines, yogurt starter, and so forth. Among them:

1. Lucy's Kitchen Shop, www.LucysKitchenShop.com (which sells superior-quality almond flour, cookbooks, a yogurt machine and starter, and other great products).

2. Digestive Wellness, www.DigestiveWellness.com (which sells kosher SCD products, nut flours, apple chips, etc.).

3. Nuts4u, www.nuts4u.com (which sells a wide variety of nut flours).

There are also many wonderful Web sites devoted to SCD, and these offer books and items for sale, as well as disseminating valuable information. The four I personally find the most helpful are:

1. www.BreakingTheViciousCycle.info – This is Elaine Gottschall's own site. I mentioned it previously when I talked about the legal/illegal list. There is an unbelievable amount of wonderful information, explanation, news, and so forth on this Web site. In spite of Elaine's passing, family and friends are maintaining the site and keeping it fully current. I browse it frequently for new information.

2. www.PecanBread.com – Earlier I mentioned Mimi, a wonderful mom whose children were immeasurably helped by SCD. Mimi and a host of other dedicated, incredibly knowledgeable mothers maintain this site and its corresponding Yahoo bulletin board. PecanBread is one of the most valuable SCD resources.

3. wwwSCDrecipe.com – This site is owned by Raman Prasad, who is the author of *Adventures in the Family Kitchen*. Raman, a former colitis sufferer, was cured via SCD and, being a wonderful cook, has collected many great recipes. His site also provides news updates, links, and other great resources.

4. www.SCDiet.org – A library of SCD information, including news, links, recipes, and so forth.

5. Finding help and support

Whether you're starting the diet immediately or easing your child into it, be sure to get involved with a parental support network. SCD is not something you can or should do alone and there are hundreds of parents out there who will be happy to help you with emotional support, recipes, and questions. As I suggested earlier, go to PecanBread's Yahoo group: http://health.groups.yahoo.com/group/PecanBread/. If there are other moms in your area who have their children on a restricted diet, talk to them. Form your own support group.

Don't make the same mistake I did by waiting to tap into the maternal information network. There is no better source of accurate, useful, potentially life-saving information than other mothers.

For example, one thing that I and my SCD-mom friends have noticed is a distinct pattern of regressions with our children on the diet. I discuss these in the next section. (Elaine told me that this is not the same for the traditional inflammatory bowel disease crowd, but it has been incredibly consistent for the autistic kids.) No one knows why these regressions occur. While you hate to see the word "regression," I strongly believe that it is always better to be prepared because you won't panic if you know there is light at the end of the regression tunnels. Anyway, the fact is that had I been doing SCD on my own, I wouldn't have been able to spot this pattern. When Alex regressed, I would have lost hope, thinking that here was yet another therapy that was failing. However, because I started the diet at the same time as a few friends did, and because our kids regressed at the same time, I was able to see that it wasn't just *my* son, for a change. I cannot describe the comfort this gave me. Without my friends' help, love, and support, Alex and I never would have made it to where we are today.

Possible Regressions

Over the two and a half years that Alex has been on the Specific Carbohydrate Diet, I have met at least 100 parents who have put their children onto the diet, and I have stayed in touch with nearly all of them. As all of our children progressed, month by month, I kept careful notes on the children's progress. It very quickly became clear that there is a distinct pattern of regressions that occur as the children heal. To date, there is no scientific explanation for it.

Not every child undergoes these regressions on SCD but it appears that most do. Before you proceed to read this section remember: **THESE REGRESSIONS ARE TEMPORARY! AS BAD AS THEY ARE WHILE YOUR CHILD IS GOING THROUGH THEM, THEY DO END! HANG IN THERE AND DON'T GIVE UP!**

Often, the worse the child's digestive problems and autistic symptoms are at the start, the worse the periods of regressions are. Alex's were indescribable, but I'm still here to tell the tale!

We have also all noted that after every period of regression, many of the children seem to show global improvement in autistic behaviors and digestive health. So the light at the end of these tunnels is pretty bright.

Initial reactions upon starting SCD

Most children undergo a distinct period of die-off at the start of the diet. Symptoms might include a regression in behavior (aggressiveness, increased hyperactivity, and self-stimulatory behaviors); poor sleep; increased obsessive behaviors; tantrums; being unfocused; maniacal laughing episodes; social withdrawal; unresponsiveness; and/or fever and vomiting. Physically, many of the children undergo a worsening of already-existing digestive troubles: children with diarrhea prior to the diet get worse diarrhea, while children with constipation get even more constipated when starting the diet. Several parents reported dark, sandy, unformed stools and also a lot of gas. Other symptoms included severe pallor of the skin, black circles around the eyes, and hiccups.

Many parents saw an enormous increase in appetite very shortly after starting the diet. The children became ravenous, eating far more than normal quantities of food.

This initial period of die-off seems to average somewhere between one and three weeks.

Regression at two to three months

Elaine mentions this regression on page five of *BTVC*. Apparently, this particular regression is common among people with IBD as well.

The vast majority of children seem to have this regression. It is both physical and behavioral and lasts up to 14 days. Symptoms of this regression can include worsening diarrhea and/or constipation; gas; bloating; poor appetite; poor sleep; decreased language; decreased eye contact; increased mouthing of objects; decreased socialization; increased self-stimulatory behaviors and hyperactivity; unexplained crying; poor focus (being "out of it"); redness around the anus; increased sensory sensitivities; increased scripting (repeating the same phrases over and over, like lines of a movie, for example), and other perseverative behaviors; tantrums; black circles around the eyes; extreme skin pallor; bumpy skin; and cold-like symptoms.

It is only after this regression that many parents start to see noticeable improvements in their children. Yes, some parents see good things almost from the start, but the majority don't until 60 to 90 days into the diet. (It is important to note that some parents have not seen improvements in their children for five or six months or more.) These improvements consist of dramatically improved bowel functioning (normal, formed, consistent bowel movements), improved attention spans, reduced self-stimulatory behaviors and hyperactivity, reduced self-abusive and aggressive behaviors, improved sleep and appetite, improved mood and sociability. The parents of children who are more verbal see increases in spontaneous language.

Regression at five months

The majority of parents see a severe regression at almost exactly the five-month anniversary. This regression lasts anywhere from seven to 21 days, and is mainly behavioral in nature. Symptoms can include increased self-stimulatory behaviors and hyperactivity; increased obsessive behaviors, perseverative play, and scripting; increased mood swings, including maniacal laughing and crying; tooth-grinding; increased self-abusive behaviors and aggression; increased defiant behavior; markedly decreased attention span; decreased social interest and social language; destructive behaviors; an enormous increase in self-directed behavior; tantrums; and itchy, white bumps on the legs. There is little worsening of bowel function and only a mild decrease of appetite.

Regression at seven months

This regression is marked by a severe worsening in bowel functioning and occurs in two phases. It appears to be finished after about five to seven days, but then seems to flare up again about two days later and lasts for another five to seven days.

Among the children in our group, all had unformed bowel movements, and some had severe diarrhea. All had enormous amounts of gas—*very* malodorous flatulence and constant burping. Several parents reported one day of fever.

The most severely affected children also have a dramatic decrease in appetite. Sleep is severely affected. Behaviorally, symptoms include a noticeable increase in self-stimulatory behaviors, dramatic increases in hyperactivity, dramatic decreases of attention span, enormous increases in obsessive behaviors and scripting, decreases in social behavior.

Regression at nine months

This is another severe and prolonged regression, lasting from seven to 21 days. One mother told me, "This was the worst regression of all. We saw behaviors we hadn't seen in a year, including hand-flapping, eye stims, weird yelping sounds, manic scripting, bad poops—the works. It peaked at a family dinner... [our daughter] spent the almost two hours running toward the lit BBQ and repeating a line from one of her books... When this passed we saw a jump in pretend play, and expressive language, and she started to laugh appropriately."

Other symptoms include severe temper tantrums, fevers, increased stimming, gas, diarrhea, bad sleep, poor appetite, and hiccups.

There also appear to be regressions at one year, 18 months, and two years. However, these are all much milder in both severity and duration than the ones occurring in the first year.

6. The question of casein

Casein is a protein found in the milk of all animals, including humans. Gluten is a protein found in many commonly used grains, including wheat, rye, spelt, and barley. Proteins are made up of long chains of amino acids, the basic building blocks for many substances in our bodies.

If digestion is working properly, the proteins we ingest are broken down into their basic amino acids, which these are subsequently used to build the proteins our body actually uses. If digestion is not working well, however, the ingested proteins may be only partially broken down into short chains of amino acids called peptides.

* * * *

Dr. Baker: *Sit down with a big box of paper clips and start hooking them together. You can make a chain in which the inside or outside loops connect and you can hook two paper clips to another to make branches. Consider the basic models that you could assemble with hundreds, even thousands, of paper clips, and you can get a sense of how starch molecules are formed from individual sugar molecules. The disassembly of a few hours' work of paper-clip chains presents the following challenge: Should you just start at one end and remove individual paper clips one at a time and put them back in the box? Or should you get a friend to start unhooking paper clips so that the chain is divided into sections while you work on the end paper clips? Digestion follows the second model. There are workers (enzymes) in your saliva and other digestive juices that specialize in dividing starch molecules into chunks, and there are others that work on the singles. Most of this work is pretty easy and goes smoothly. When it comes to final units that consist of just two paper clips (disaccharides), your enzymes encounter a uniquely resistant bond requiring a special enzymatic* knack. *When you have any kind of digestive upset, your disaccharide enzymes (disaccharidases) may become temporarily impaired. Normally these enzymes bounce back when you recover. But what happens when the sugars that go undigested slip through to feed a few germs that normally inhabit your digestive tract? Those germs may feast and produce toxins that injure you in ways that reduce disaccharidase production. Voila! The start of a vicious cycle.*

* * * *

In a person with a damaged intestinal wall, these peptides leak into the body and bloodstream. In the case of poorly digested casein and gluten, the peptides caseomorphin and gluteomorphin are formed and, as they strongly resemble opiates (such as opium and heroine) that affect our endorphin receptors, these peptides can cause a literal intoxication.

About 40 to 60% of children on the autism spectrum respond positively to the removal of casein and gluten from their diets. However, many, like Alex, show no improvements at all. What differentiates a responder from a non-responder is not known. More importantly, even those children who do respond to a casein-/gluten-free (GFCF) diet will usually respond even better to SCD.

There is one important difference to note between SCD and the GF diet: GF is a diet for life. Because the removal of these proteins does not result in the healing of the damaged walls of the intestines, the leaky gut and poor digestion remain. Yes, in some children the removal of these offending substances may make enough difference (between decreasing the intoxicating peptides and reducing the hyperinflammatory response caused by these "enemy" particles entering the body) to result in at least partial, and sometimes a full, cure. However, gluten-free does not heal. SCD, on the other hand, by shifting the balance of the gut flora and by starving the bacteria that are causing the damage, eventually leads to a healthy digestive tract. After a varying period of time on SCD (as I discuss later in this chapter), all children should be able to eat a totally normal diet (except for foods to which they have a severe allergy).

This brings me to the question of the homemade yogurt. Most experts agree that there is no better way of getting good bacteria into the intestine than via cultured milk (yogurt) and other cultured foods. After the gut has some time to heal on SCD, even the most casein-sensitive children demonstrate an ability to tolerate the protein. Moreover, in many cases, the yogurt dramatically improves bowel functioning. In many higher-functioning children, immediate improvements in socialization, language, and imaginative play have been seen.

It is a wise idea to avoid all casein for at least three months (for non-casein responders) and for at least six months if your child has demonstrated improvement from casein removal in the past. The introduction of yogurt early in the diet can result in a severe regression. Don't take that risk.

Another caution: Start *very* slowly, at a quarter-teaspoon per day or every other day, depending on how well the first dose is tolerated. Build up slowly, over the course of weeks.

I still find it remarkable that, after a period of time on SCD, even children who went from frankly autistic to nearly neurotypical following the removal of casein and gluten are now consuming a full cup of yogurt every day and some are now also eating cheese with no ill effect. What greater proof can there be of SCD's power to heal?

I mix Alex's yogurt with honey and fruit. (I vary it with ripe bananas, mangos, papayas, peaches, blueberries, or any mixture thereof.) His brother, my nine-year-old typically developing son Liam loves it, and it has become one of his absolute favorite desserts. Most kids do love it. I know of very few cases of a child who has objected to eating the yogurt.

7. Other important information to know before starting the diet

You are now familiar with how SCD works. By starving the bad gut flora of nutrients (undigested sugars and starches), the diet starves them to death. When yeast dies, it causes what is known as a Heximer reaction, a flood of bad toxins into the body, also known as die-off. (I always imagine yeast looking sort of like a dandelion that's reached its seeding stage: you blow on it and those fluffy little white seeds explode all over.) This die-off reaction occurs with both yeast and, it appears, bacteria as well.

Not all people on SCD experience a period of initial die-off, but many—if not most—do. It can be *very* difficult to get through, but persevere you must. It is often the children who undergo the worst regressions who benefit the most from SCD (although this is certainly not always the case).

What does this die-off look like? To briefly summarize: children who have diarrhea get severely worse diarrhea (see Chapter One). Children who have constipation often become more severely constipated. There can be vomiting, fevers, cold-like symptoms, gas, bloating, poor appetite, and rashes. Autistic symptoms can get dramatically worse. This initial die-off can last anywhere from just a few days to months, as in Alex's case. He, however, was unusual—not a surprise though, when you consider the severity of his gut symptoms.

You must do everything you can to support your child through this potentially difficult period. If your child has chronic diarrhea, you will want to be very careful about which foods you use at the start of the diet. Certain foods are very difficult for some people to digest and can exacerbate diarrhea. Peel all fruits and vegetables and cook them. Skins are inflammatory. Cooking fibrous foods makes them easier to digest. Limit nuts and use only well-ground (not whole) ones. PecanBread.com recommends an "intro diet" for children with more severe digestive issues. I didn't do this with Alex only because I started the diet within three hours of reading Elaine's book and hadn't yet realized that there was help on the Internet. I never heard of the intro diet when I started SCD. I wish I had, in retrospect, because it might have helped alleviate the worst of those early incredibly severe symptoms.

The intro diet consists of foods like chicken broth with chunks of cooked (and peeled) carrots and chicken; roasted chicken and turkey; beef broth; ground beef (either in the broth or as hamburger); eggs; and homemade jello. As you can see, all the foods are *very* easy to digest, and carrots are wonderful for helping with diarrhea.

If your child has chronic constipation, the intro diet couldn't hurt, but as it is low in fiber (since fiber is more difficult to digest), it could worsen constipation. If this is an issue, consider adding more fruits and vegetables.

Another warning: be careful of extremely difficult-to-digest vegetables like things in the cabbage family. Very hard-to-digest foods will worsen bloating and gas and make your child *really* uncomfortable. Foods to avoid include cabbage, broccoli, cauliflower, broccoli rabe, and brussels sprouts. Also, foods like beans and seeds should not be eaten for quite some time. (I didn't use any for almost 18 months with Alex because his gas and bloating were so severe.)

A few other tips:

1. I noticed that whole nuts, even 18 months or more into the diet,

caused Alex's stools to loosen. Without being too graphic, it was obvious that he was having difficulty digesting them. He tolerates all baked goods well but the whole nuts seem to be problematic and this is not at all unusual.

2. During periods of regression, it can never hurt to go back to the intro diet for a few days. Notice that it's not unlike the foods you would eat if you were sick—for good reason.

3. If your child appears to have a flare-up of yeasty behaviors—a red ring around the anus, eczema, maniacal laughing (although this can also be caused by bacterial overgrowth), moodiness, red ears and/or cheeks, etc.—you might want to cut out foods high in monosaccharide sugars. Until these symptoms subside, stay away from honey, for example. Also, the best fruit to use is pears, as it appears that even the children with the worst gut dysbiosis tolerate pears well.

Finally, there is one very important issue to discuss before you start the diet. Because of severe die-off that can occur at the start, many children lose weight at first. As they start to feel better, however, they will eat more, and they will regain any weight they lost, plus put on some good, healthy pounds. To date, Alex has gained about 20 pounds in two years! I should also mention that because SCD is such a naturally balanced and healthy diet, it is also good for losing weight if that is necessary. If the wish is to drop pounds, simply restrict the amount of nuts consumed.

* * * *

Dr. Baker: *The term "die-off" refers to symptoms evoked by the release of toxic substances associated with the death of germs. The original model for the concept derived from the reaction of patients with syphilis to early treatments that caused the death of the syphilis germs and—in the process—triggered the transient appearance of symptoms of toxicity. Similarly, when large doses of antifungal medicines such as nystatin were used to treat individuals who had developed a sensitivity to yeast germs growing in abnormal numbers or in abnormal parts of the digestive tract, some patients experienced a temporary exacerbation of many of their symptoms. The capacity of different antifungal medicines to evoke identical reactions—and the power of activated charcoal to quench the reaction by absorbing the toxins—led to the notion that toxins released with the death of the targeted organisms were the cause of the negative symptoms. Parents observing this connection in their children have tended to* *expand the use of the term "die-off" beyond its original meaning and apply it to any regression or constellation of symptoms associated with a change that might affect gut flora.*

* * * *

8. Misconceptions about SCD

1. First and foremost, SCD is *not* a low-carbohydrate diet. Unlike the Atkins diet, which limits the amount of carbohydrates consumed each day, SCD limits only the *type* of carbohydrates eaten, not the amounts. Be sure to give your child plenty of fruits and vegetables every day, as well as legal fruit juices and honey (assuming there is no significant yeast issue).

When the body is deprived of carbohydrates (which provide glucose, the body's energy source), it will begin to break down stored fats to get the required energy to operate. When fats are broken down, ketones are released, which make the blood acidic. For multiple reasons this is extremely unhealthy. As bad gut flora also tend to cause the blood to be acidic, it is especially important in children with autism to avoid ketosis. It is absolutely vital that you find ways of getting fruits and vegetables into your child several times per day.

* * * *

Dr. Baker: *When we burn fat with a shortage of carbohydrate, the "smoke" from the fat is not the normal combination of just water and carbon dioxide but contains incompletely metabolized fat in the form of ketones. These volatile compounds produce a sweet or fruity aroma on the breath; it is not unusual to find it in children who are just plain very hungry or sick. People who do a very-low-carbohydrate diet, such as the Atkins diet, check their urine to see if they are producing ketones (a sign that they are being strict with their diet). Diabetics, who cannot usher their blood sugar from the bloodstream into cells, also produce ketones in their urine as a sign of poor control of their diabetes. Ketones on the breath or in the urine are not a good thing for our kids doing SCD because they indicate an overly short supply of carbohydrates. It may, however, be hard to avoid this occasionally as you are learning to adjust the diet—assuring a sufficiency of fruit and vegetables.*

* * * *

2. "There's nothing to use as reinforcers for my child." There are many delicious and healthy foods for your kids to eat as primary reinforcers. Cookies, cakes, chips... there's never a reason for anyone to feel deprived. I have a friend who made her daughter an Elmo cake for her birthday. She cooked strawberries and used the juice to color the icing made from the recipe in *BTVC*. If you use your imagination, get help from other moms with more experience, and use the resources I've provided above, you can recreate many, if not all, of your child's favorite foods in an SCD-legal form.

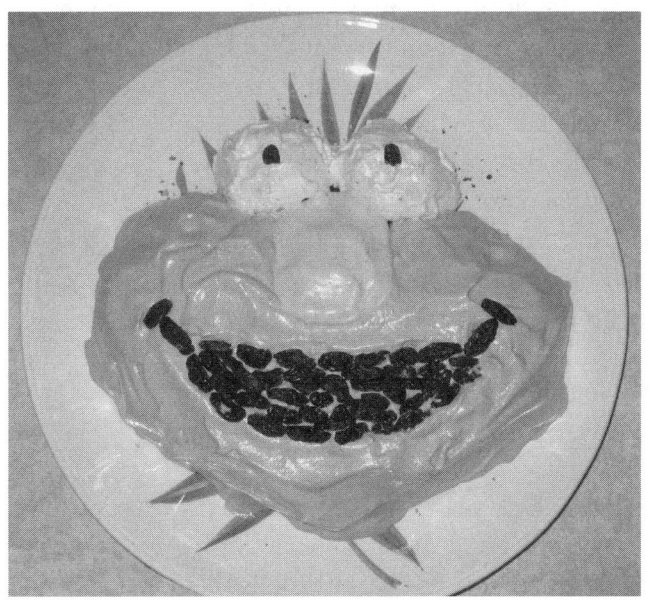

3. Thirdly, if your kids have food allergies—even to nuts—SCD is still a possibility. Granted, it's not easy. But there are plenty of moms out there doing it right now. Instead of using nut flours, they use pumpkin seed flour or bean flours. Again, no matter what the dietary restriction, SCD is manageable.

9. When you're really ready to start

Consider yourself ready to start when you've:

1. Set up your kitchen binder (with the list of legal/illegal foods in it and whatever recipes you found on the Internet or got from friends).

2. Created your substitutions list.

3. Bought the necessary groceries.

4. Worked on transitioning your child if necessary.

5. Set up your account with Yahoo groups and joined PecanBread.

One other good idea before you officially declare it 100% SCD-legal day: make sure you have plenty of activated charcoal in the house. Activated charcoal is available in any pharmacy, usually in the first aid section. It's good to have it in the house anyway, as it is often used in poison control. It will absorb anything it comes into contact with, so if there's a burst of toxins from die-off, it will make your child much more comfortable. (Beware: it does turn bowel movements black!) It usually comes in capsule form, so if your child can't swallow pills, empty the capsules into juice or water, in an opaque sippy cup. It will turn the liquid black, so children don't like it if they see it. However, it has no taste, so it's not hard to get them to take it. I empty Alex's into a small medicine cup and use a syringe to get it into him. He will actually ask for it sometimes if he needs it.

Please note: because charcoal will absorb anything, do not give it within an hour either side of medicine or supplements!

10. Tailoring the diet to your child's specific needs

I have many friends who have found it necessary (because of allergies, food intolerances, high yeast levels, and so forth) to tailor the diet to meet their children's individual dietary restrictions or particular biochemical needs. Remember that on SCD, many foods that are not initially tolerated will be reintroduced after the gut has some time to heal. However, with some kids who have severe allergies, for example, this may be a long time in coming. And nut allergies don't go away. My friend Heather has a little boy with the worst allergies I have ever seen (see Heather's and Aidan's story in Chapter Five). Before SCD, he would go into anaphylactic shock frequently, requiring shots of epinephrine to get his airway open. The amount of effort Heather has had to put into getting her son onto SCD is extraordinary, considering the number of foods he cannot eat. Once a month Heather's husband drives three hours each way to a game farm to stock up on meats their child can eat, like bear. His grain allergies are so severe that he reacted even to chicken that was corn-fed. He will die if he eats a nut and can tolerate only a limited selection of fruit (as long as it is absolutely fresh, with no trace of mold on the skins), very few vegetables, and certain proteins. However, Heather would be the first to say that the effort of sorting out a way to keep him on SCD has been worth every minute of extra work. In the two years since she started SCD, her son has gone from a three-and-a-half-year-old boy who had to be home-schooled in an environmentally controlled setting to essentially a normally developing child, attending a local kindergarten independently. I have had lengthy conversations with him on topics as esoteric as Egyptian sarcophagi. When my parents met him, my father took me aside and whispered, "Are you trying to tell me that this child was autistic?!"

Stories like this lead me back to that mantra I've developed over the years: NO MERCY. If Heather can keep her child on this diet no matter what, if I can do it with my son trying to destroy himself and our house—so can you.

11. What if it's not working?

As all of us in the world of autism know, unfortunately, nothing is going to work for every child. There's just too much variability among the children who fall under the autism umbrella. Even if you don't see improvement in your child from SCD, the good news is that it can't hurt to have tried it. The diet is incredibly healthful and you've done nothing but feed your child exceptionally nutrient-rich, wholesome foods.

However, there are other possibilities to consider before declaring your child an SCD non-responder.

A. Have you done the diet long enough? SCD is not a fast heal but a slow and gradual process. As I said earlier, some children do respond almost immediately but most don't, and some children take many months to show beneficial effects. I know of one child, Eric (whose story is told in Chapter Five), who took almost a full year to show improvement. Things also can be made more complex by potential bad reactions to other treatments you're trying. Certainly, if you've committed to giving SCD a real try, you need to start with the idea that you'll be giving it a fair trial for at least six months, preferably a year.

B. Does your child have food intolerances about which you are unaware? In Alex's case, for example, even though cashews were legal, he just couldn't tolerate them. Only careful observation on your part can sort this out.

C. Are you giving any illegal foods by accident? Check your menus and ingredients. Some children can tolerate small amounts of illegals, but some can't. If you've "cheated" and have been using store-bought ketchup thinking that a smidge of sugar won't matter, you might have to think again. Also, be very careful about illegals in supplements (until you can show that the relatively trivial amounts of starches, or even sugars, in capsules or tablets are not associated with negative symptoms)!

D. Are you feeding your child foods that are hard to digest? Aberrant gut bacteria cause massive amounts of gas in the intestines. It's not a great idea then, at least until your child's had plenty of time to heal, to feed her foods like broccoli, cauliflower, beans, and so forth, whose high-fiber content can cause gas in some people. Again, check your list of current foods. You may have to pull out anything that is extremely fibrous. Also, you may have to go back to peeling and cooking all fruit and vegetables for some time.

E. Is there something else going on? As I discussed in the section on tailoring the diet, it is possible that your child not only needs the SCD diet, but also needs to avoid foods containing certain natural substances. Again, because there is no one-size-fits-all in the world of autism, it's up to you, through careful observation, to figure out if there are other foods you need to avoid.

12. When can I stop?!

Elaine Gottschall recommended continuing with SCD until the patient has been symptom-free for at least a year. It's a good rule of thumb because, in fact, at this point no one knows for sure. I have several friends now whose children were on a strict SCD diet for two years and who then have ventured to give small amounts of illegal foods. To date, none has reported any adverse affects. However, I do want to note that their children were far less affected than Alex in terms of both gastrointestinal illness and autistic symptoms. My son will be on SCD for several years more. While he has formed bowel movements on most days, has gas and bloating only infrequently, and never vomits unless he's sick, he still has a poor appetite on and off, occasional soft and grainy stools, and so forth, which indicate to me that we still have a lot of healing to do. When to end strict adherence to the diet will have to be a decision you make based on your parental instinct: Is your child healed? Has progress stopped? If you decide that the time has come, go slowly and cautiously. Remember, if your child has an adverse reaction to the reintroduction of illegal foods, you can always go back onto SCD. It's always there, waiting to help, if necessary!

I want to conclude this chapter with a little section from my speech at the Boston DAN! conference in April 2005:

> *Make Alex's sickness have meaning. Please—learn from my experience and my mistakes. Nothing else you do is going to work if your child's digestion isn't working right. For seven and a half years I did everything there was out there, from healers to medications, and from crystals to vitamins—but nothing ever made a difference until I put him on SCD.*
>
> *Over these last 18 months I have had the blessing of watching children of all ages and functioning levels make dramatic improvements on SCD. Even children who had no overt gastrointestinal symptoms have done incredibly well, in terms of improved language, imaginative play, and socialization. So now I have developed a "no mercy" policy about this.*
>
> *I don't want to hear from any of you that all your child eats is french fries, pretzels and potato chips. What do you think Alex ate? I don't want to hear that your children will starve rather than eat a piece of chicken. It took me years of miserable hard work, but I got Alex to eat chicken, steak, fruit, and vegetables. If our children can do without McDonald's french fries, so can yours. I have no pity. Yes, changing your child's diet is hard. But I'm telling you now, with nine years of experience behind me, having a profoundly sick and autistic child is a hell of a lot harder.*
>
> **As I said, I have no mercy. There are no excuses.**

CHAPTER V

From the Mouths of Mothers

The following chapter contains stories from real moms with kids on the autism spectrum whose lives have been changed by SCD. Elaine had hundreds of such testimonials in her files. And I have scores of friends now with children on SCD. I have had the incredible experience and blessing of watching children heal from a close-up view. There is nothing in the world more wonderful than seeing a child get well.

And to make a child get well, there is nothing better than SCD.

Perhaps that is the most amazing thing about the Specific Carbohydrate Diet. It doesn't just help kids like Alex, the low-functioning, severely sick kids. I have witnessed its ability to help people of every age, from infants to adults, from kids with severe gut problems to kids with no discernable gut issues at all. Of course, *how* it helps the kids varies in some ways. But there is also continuity throughout the stories: there are always improvements in health and digestive function, and also possibly increased language. Certainly there is improved awareness and sociability. With the high-functioning kids, moms tell me about major developmental leaps in imagination. The list goes on. In fact, I'll step aside now and let these moms tell you their own stories.

* * * *

1. Zachary's Story, by Candace Bender, R.N.

At seven pounds, three and a half ounces, he was the most beautiful boy I had ever seen. I delivered him naturally. Little did I know that the pain of childbirth would never come close to the pain and suffering we would soon experience.

It was a fairytale, a happily-ever-after kind of life for the first 15 months. The kind of things that make parents proud. Walking, talking, playing ball, and annoying his big sister were all on Zachary's agenda. He was perfect. I wanted to protect him from everything. We never missed a check-up and always had his vaccinations up to date.

In January of 2002, all of that changed. Zachary received his first MMR. Ten days later he was a different child. He broke out in a rash, spiked a high fever, and screamed inconsolably for days. The doctor's office said, "Give him Tylenol and call if he gets worse."

Call if he gets worse! How about, call if he loses eye contact, call if he doesn't respond to his name, call if he won't play with his toys anymore, call if he engages in repetitive activities for hours on end, or call if he doesn't seem to recognize his own mother.

Over the next two years, we did a lot of calling. Zachary was evaluated by family doctors, pediatricians, speech therapists, behavior specialists, occupational therapists, psychiatrists, pediatric neurologists, gastroenterologists, and doctors who specialize in the treatment of autism.

Yes, Zachary was autistic. My beautiful, perfect child had retreated into his own personal hell and we didn't know how to get him back. As a matter of fact, everything we tried seemed to push him deeper and further out of reach. Zachary lost all language, began to engage is self-stimulatory activities, and became self-injurious. He developed chronic diarrhea and a bloated belly, and vomited two or three times a day. He was thin, gaunt, and had dark circles under his eyes. He slept only two to four hours a night.

In July of 2004, we consulted a gastroenterologist and learned that Zachary had esophagitis, gastritis, duodenitis with duodenal erosions (ulcers), ileitis with marked lymphonodular hyperplasia, and mild colitis with diffuse lymphoid hyperplasia throughout the colon. Zachary was immediately placed on steroids to combat the inflammation in his gut. The vomiting stopped overnight, but not much else changed. We tried no less than seven different drugs to heal his gut without success.

Zachary spent most of his day in misery. Lost in his own world, and unable to tell anyone what was wrong, he would spend hours beating his head against the floor, biting his flesh, and throwing his body against anything hard enough to cause pain. It would happen without warning. He would double over, drop to his knees, and start beating his forehead against the floor so hard that it caused bruising and swelling. Then he would roll over on his back and slam the back of his head against the floor while biting his hands and forearms. After a while he began to develop scarring on his wrists from the constant biting. It was a permanent reminder of the agony he experienced. As if this wasn't bad enough, he would slam his forearms against the edge of our kitchen table or bite the furniture so hard I was sure he would crack a tooth. I still have tooth marks in my butcher block that make me cringe every time I see them. To a parent, it was unbearable to watch. The only way to keep him from hurting himself was to physically restrain him. This often resulted in my being rewarded with a swollen lip, a bruised cheek, or multiple bite marks.

We tried everything: vitamins, minerals, dietary changes, and even antipsychotic medication. Nothing worked. He was having six to eight liquid stools a day with undigested food coming out of him. His belly was distended with gas and his face was round and bloated from the steroids.

In December 2004, Zachary's gastroenterologist recommended I call a mother whose child had similar problems and made remarkable progress on a special diet. That night I called Judy. She was sympathetic, reassuring, and more motivating than anyone I had talked to. Suddenly, I didn't feel so alone. If her son could improve on the Specific Carbohydrate Diet, so could mine.

It was Christmas Eve when I made the big step. I couldn't stand to watch my son suffer another day. I threw out practically everything in the kitchen and started from scratch. It was my Christmas gift to him.

He was so sick that he ate no solid food for three days. Then, slowly but surely, he began to come around. He started to enjoy his SCD food, and within a week his appetite was back. He was eating nutritious, well-balanced meals.

Within five months of starting the SCD, Zachary was off the steroids, off his antipsychotic medication, and sleeping through the night. Within

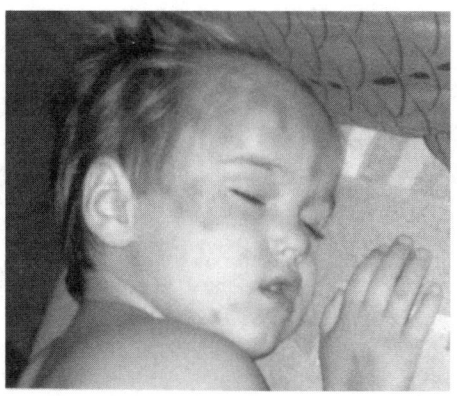

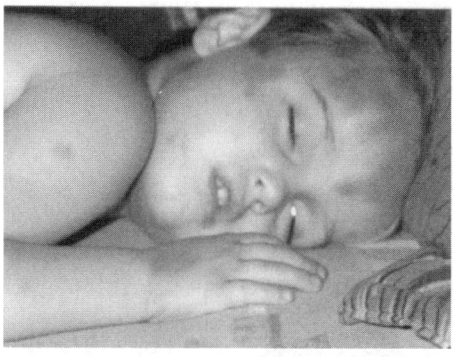

Zachary after 48-hour hospital admission
for abdominal pain, September 2004

ten months, he was having two to three formed bowel movements a day and had gained a few pounds.

Today, Zachary eats three meals a day and hasn't vomited once since starting the SCD. His belly is flat, the pain is gone, and the self-injurious behavior is just a bad memory. He attends preschool and a playgroup five days a week. His teachers and therapists are amazed by his transformation. They are finally able to teach him something. He is playing with toys and beginning to interact with his peers. He communicates through sign language and picture exchange, and lately he's starting to say a few words. The Specific Carbohydrate Diet didn't cure Zachary's autism, but it certainly made him more receptive to biomedical and educational interventions. For the first time in years, my son is able to learn, laugh, and play.

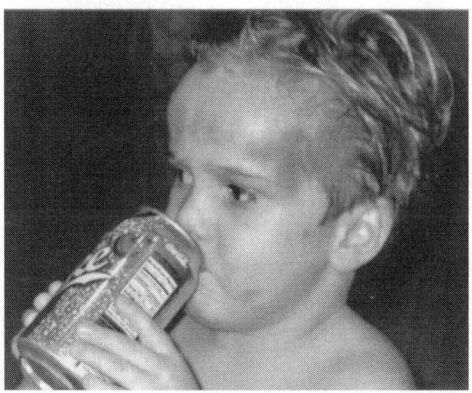

Christmas 2004, age two years, four months—
This is why we started the Specific Carbohydrate Diet

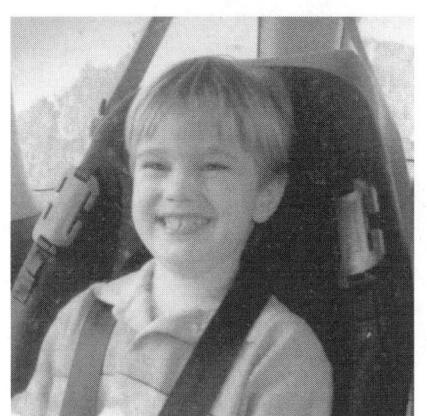 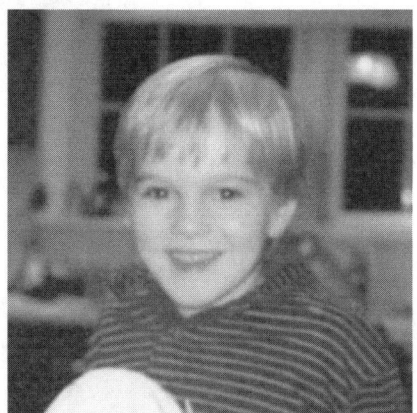

Zachary six months after starting the SCD (left), and today (right)

2. Jack and Jay, by Jean Loftus, M.D.

Jack, our precious first-born child, was a calm, content baby for about two weeks. Thereafter, he was perpetually colicky for about three years. At two months, when other infants were offering social smiles, we could seldom get Jack to look at us. Instead, he mostly looked through us. Over the next three years, he sometimes smiled, giggled, and engaged with us, although he was more often aloof, serious, intense, and task-oriented. He had a large vocabulary by the age of two, but we were the only ones who could understand him, as his articulation was poor. He typically looked away from the person to whom he spoke, even when he was asking a question. He knew his name but usually did not turn or respond to it. He showed no imaginary play and did not imitate us.

Around the age of two, he contracted rotavirus, a common childhood viral illness that causes vomiting and diarrhea. His GI tract never seemed to recover completely, as he continued to have frequent pasty yellow stools, which we later learned were a result of yeast overgrowth. Around this time he developed sleep problems and awakened in the night, confused and unable to be calmed. Soon he had problems getting to sleep, and then had difficulty taking naps. As a result of his sleep deprivation, he became even more whiny, demanding, unhappy, and discontent. He started having sensory problems, such that he could not tolerate lotions (moisturizing lotion or sunscreen). He cried and screamed as though we were abusing him each time we applied them. Each time he fell, he screamed as though it was a major injury. He didn't like being tickled, and sometimes did not like being touched. Unlike other toddlers and preschoolers, he rarely showed emotion when we came home or left for work. We would say goodbye, but he would ignore us. We convinced ourselves that this was just his way of dealing with our departure. By the age of two and a half, he became regularly hyperactive: he was constantly jumping, throwing, screaming, and destroying. Time-outs had no effect on him.

No longer was I willing to live in denial, hiding behind the comfort that Jack did occasionally smile and engage with us. I abandoned the rationalization that all kids are different, along with the expectation that he would grow out of it. So my husband Jim and I sought evaluation at the prestigious children's hospital in our city. The physician who evaluated Jack was the chairperson of the Division of Developmental Disabilities and told us that Jack had some autistic tendencies, but was not frankly autistic. Had Jack attempted to speak less, then he would have met the ADOS criteria for autism. Imagine our surprise when she then told us to "wait and see if he grows out of it."

Unwilling to accept this advice, we took matters into our own hands. We started numerous vitamins, minerals, and supplements in accordance with the recommendations of DAN! Nothing helped. We started the GFCF diet (gluten- and casein-free diet), but it made Jack worse, not better. Jack's hyperactive behavior escalated into manic behavior. He had spontaneous outbursts of maniacal laughter, shrieking in public, and echolalia (repeating our words). His sleep worsened, as did his stools. Prior to starting GFCF, Jack had three food sensitivities. After six months of GFCF, Jack had developed 31 food sensitivities.

It became evident only in retrospect why Jack worsened on GFCF. A number of the foods that are forbidden on GFCF, such as milk products and wheat products, have substitutes that are based on potatoes and rice. For example, we switched Jack from milk to a potato-based beverage. In doing so, we markedly increased his daily intake of complex carbohydrates. In Jack, as in many children who have dysbiosis, complex carbohydrates are not broken down and absorbed. They remain instead in the lumen of the gut and are available to nourish yeast and unfavorable bacteria (dysbiosis), thus making the GI problem worse. Jack's problem was so severe that months of prescription antifungal medications at high doses failed to improve his yeast issues while on GFCF. Yet, our first DAN! physician kept suggesting more.

As physicians, we knew that giving more of the same in larger doses was not the answer, but we did not know what the answer was. It was around this time that Jim attended the spring 2005 DAN! conference in Boston, where he heard Judy speak about the Specific Carbohydrate Diet. We started SCD shortly thereafter, in May 2005, at about the time Jack turned three.

Jack had an initial die-off, followed by resolution of all of his maniacal behaviors within two weeks. More strikingly, he developed excellent eye contact during the same period. Imagine how our thinking changed as we, two physicians, witnessed our son being healed by diet, not antifungals or antibiotics.

Meanwhile, Jay, our precious second-born child, who is Jack's younger brother by two years, started having problems. In the midst of Jack's battle with yeast and manic behavior, we noticed that Jay was showing early signs of dysbiosis and immune system dysregulation. Although Jay had been a smiling happy baby, he had developed eczema at six months and fifth disease (a common viral illness) at nine months. Thereafter, he became colicky. I kept thinking it would resolve, but it did not. It got worse when we switched him from formula to milk at 12 months. Then sleep disturbances started. Then we saw yellow pasty stools. Then he stopped pointing and stopped saying some words. Jay was tested and was found to have over 20 food sensitivities, severe dysbiosis, and a genetic predisposition to ASD by way of several deficient enzymes. Eager to treat Jay aggressively, and having seen Jack's impressive response to SCD, we started Jay on SCD in July 2005, at the age of 15 months. Within two weeks, he was sleeping, happy, pointing, and had twenty new words and five animal sounds. We withheld his MMR vaccine with the plan to give it to him after the age of three as separate vaccinations.

Prior to starting Jack on SCD, we had abandoned our long-standing intention of sending him to Montessori preschool in fall 2005. Our local public school system evaluated Jack, deemed him developmentally delayed due to behavior and social problems, and accepted him into a preschool program for children with special needs. Within three months of starting SCD, Jack made great gains. Even though he still had problems with hyperactivity and inattention, we felt he could succeed in Montessori school, and we chose that route. His first few months were not pretty. Other kids could sit still and listen; Jack usually could not. His five-month regression was notably the most difficult time.

SCD was the first and most important step we have taken toward curing our sons. And it was with intense vigilance that we followed the diet and anticipated regressions. So, when regressions failed to occur after six months for Jack—and never came for Jay—we started to wonder. We also noted failure to continue to improve after this point. And we continued to be plagued with dysbiosis. With ongoing problems despite SCD, another mom suggested to me that we should consider the Low Oxalate Diet (LOD). At this time, Jack had been on SCD for nine months and Jay had been on SCD for eight months. The principles of LOD made sense, so we maintained SCD and modified it by removing high-oxalate foods, such as most nuts and a few other foods. Both boys had an immediate die-off and significant improvement.

Although Jack and Jay did not consume huge amounts of nuts, we learned from this that in some children, regular nut consumption over several months can sometimes cause problems, such as oxalate issues.

As of this writing in May 2006, Jack has now been on SCD for 11 months. Jack's behavior has improved along with his stools. He has gone from having five bowel movements each day to one or two. They are mostly formed. His number of food sensitivities has decreased form 31 to 20. Jack now has some days in which he is neurotypical... and even neuro-ideal, such that his behavior and social interactions are truly amazing for any three-year-old. He is often charming, engaging, sensitive, responsive, and interactive. His episodes of hyperactivity are becoming fewer and milder. His whininess, sleep, speech, and sensory integration all improved. He is now consistently happy for the first time. He even likes being tickled. And he frequently tells me about his imaginary pet, Baby Sharptooth, a dinosaur who fits in the palm of his hand. This progress did not come easily or smoothly, as the hallmark of SCD is fluctuating improvement mixed with (usually) predictable regressions.

Jay has had more ups and downs than Jack. His dysbiosis initially improved on SCD, but worsened markedly during his third and fourth months. He had a notable major regression lasting four months, which improved after we converted him to SCD/LOD. Now he is ten months into SCD, but still having problems with dysbiosis. He is generally happy, pointing, saying new words, and smiling at everyone. His speech is within normal range for his age. He is sleeping without interruption most nights. Jay had twenty food sensitivities when he started SCD, but only ten after he had been on SCD for six months. His allergies to peanuts, peas, carrots, and beef (among other foods) resolved. On the downside, Jay has developed two new food allergies while on the diet. This is unusual for children on SCD, as they typically resolve food allergies while on the diet, rather than acquire them. Although this is a concern and disappointment, I suspect that his food allergies might be much worse had we not started SCD.

SCD is not our endpoint; it is just the beginning. It served as a foundation upon which we built the rest of the boys' treatment plans, including detoxification and antiviral medication (for Jack). Without SCD, we would undoubtedly still be losing the battle against dysbiosis. I am convinced that Jack would still have the social and behavioral problems he had prior to SCD, and I shudder to think where Jay might be. Thank you, Judy, for spreading the word about SCD and for being there to help us with our questions and concerns!

3. Amanda's Story

In September of 2002, my two-and-a-half-year-old daughter Amanda was diagnosed with PDD or regressive autism. This beautiful and intelligent little girl who, at her one-year check-up, was able to read all the letters on the eye chart, knew all of her numbers and colors, and was speaking in two-word sentences at 16 months, had by the age of two lost all of her language except for the word "up." Even worse, she had absolutely no eye contact, spun in circles, and crossed her eyes constantly—a horrible sight.

Amanda craved milk so much that she was drinking eight to ten cups of it a day, and she suffered from chronic diarrhea.

* * * *

Dr. Baker: *When I take a medical history from any patient with a chronic health problem, the following question is very helpful: "Is there any food that you crave or that you tend to eat on a daily basis?" Naturally, some habitual eating is just that, a habit. On the other hand, repetitive eating and craving may indicate intolerance to a food. There is a connection among craving and addiction and allergy. For example, if I ask a person with, say, chronic joint pain, "If you were asked to change your diet for a week or so to see if you might get relief of your pain, is there any particular food that you'd really miss?" and the person replies, "Potatoes," then potato moves to the top of the list of foods I would suspect as an allergic cause of the joint pain. Sugar and carbohydrate craving is another matter. Habitual eating of sugars and starches tends, in itself, to reinforce cravings for them. Individuals with yeast problems develop particularly intense sugar and starch cravings as well as strong preferences for yeasty bread, vinegar, wine, beer and other products of yeast fermentation. Salt craving is different, and represents a true indication of an unmet need, which may be caused by simply not getting enough salt, but may be an indication of an unmet need for other minerals, particularly magnesium. Abnormal salt losses associated with adrenal insufficiency are associated with salt craving, which is reflective of a very sensitive mechanism for regulation of sufficiency of sodium and chloride in the blood. The quest for salt in regions far from the ocean was a major factor in human migration and settlement in our early history.*

* * * *

When Amanda was a little over three years old, we started her on the gluten-free, casein-free diet (GFCF), and at first we saw good things from it. She was much calmer and more socially connected, and with the help of speech and ABA therapy, she was gaining some of her words back. After about four months of GFCF, though, it wouldn't be an exaggeration to say that we had descended into a nightmare. Amanda craved rice in all its forms—cooked rice, rice cakes, rice puffs. She wouldn't eat any kind of meat or vegetables, and would only occasionally eat an apple or a handful of grapes. Obviously, this was far from a healthy diet for a three-and-a-half-year-old. The worst part of it was that all the old stims had come back and her language became repetitive. She would constantly script lines from *Winnie the Pooh* or *Sleeping Beauty* all day long. Never a good sleeper, by that September Amanda was only sleeping three or four hours a night. Unfortunately, it was rarely the same three or four hours that her five-month-old sister slept. That summer of 2003, my husband and I were each getting only an hour or two of sleep a night as Amanda spun faster and faster out of control. Something had to give.

Looking for answers, I joined the Yahoo GFCF discussion group. One day a mother, to whom I will be forever grateful, posted the address of the Web site for a diet called the Specific Carbohydrate Diet (SCD). On September 22, I logged onto www.BreakingTheViciousCycle.info and read the incredible story of Elaine Gottschall and how she saved her daughter's life through SCD. That night I went through my kitchen and threw out all of the "illegal" foods—rice, potatoes, GFCF pretzels—they all had to go. The next day I bought some almond flour, made Amanda some SCD muffins, and I've been baking ever since!

Our journey on SCD has been far from easy. On the second day of not eating any complex carbohydrates, Amanda was extremely sick, vomiting green liquid and running a fever of about 103°F. But for the first time in over two years, she sat on my lap and let me read books to her. Prior to SCD, she was so hyperactive that she couldn't sit still for more than a second or two. Her eye contact improved and she started being more affectionate, giving her baby sister hugs and kisses. About a week into the diet, I called my friend Judy and told her about SCD. Judy had been Amanda's shadow at her nursery school, and I knew that she also had a child who was vaccine-injured. Judy immediately started Alex on SCD and during those first few weeks Judy and I were each other's support system. We constantly compared notes, and when Amanda had a massive behavioral and intestinal regression at about 21 days into the diet, I was able to tell Judy about it so that she would be prepared when Alex hit the regression a week later.

At just about the two-month mark, Amanda hit what we later realized was going to be the second in a series of these regressions. Seemingly out of nowhere, Amanda had started stimming and scripting out of control again, and her poops were a mess. I sat down at my kitchen table, looked around at all the dirty pots, pans, and cupcake tins, and just starting bawling. I hated cooking, I hated cleaning up after cooking, and quite frankly, at that point I asked myself -- Who needs this? I just wanted to be normal like other people, and go out to dinner with my kids or go to the McDonald's drive-thru and get those gluten-free french fries.

Thank goodness for Judy! She gave me the mother of all pep talks, and my husband and I decided to stick with the diet. At the three-month mark, Amanda potty trained, and a month later she started having "trophies"—perfectly formed poops. Her scripting drastically decreased, and we started to see some pretend play and increased interaction with her little sister. Regressions at five, seven, nine, twelve, eighteen, and twenty-four months followed. Amanda's worst regression of all was at the nine-month mark. It was so bad that I once again considered giving up on SCD, because it seemed like she was having a reaction to every food I gave her. However, once it passed she made another big leap in expressive and receptive language.

* * * *

Dr. Baker: *Children grow in leaps. Development in childhood—and into adult life—does not go in a smooth line. The changes we associate with developmental progress form a wavy line, which, if illustrated graphically, would rise across the page as a sequence of ups and downs. Downs? Yes, there is a consistent pattern of dis-integration that precedes the integration of skills when a developmental leap occurs. Regressions that precede developmental leaps can be confusing when they are mapped against the effects of other stresses, such as those associated with starting or stopping various treatments. The healing curve has the same configuration as the waves of development, so that as a child or an adult recovers from an illness, the progress is associated with ups and downs. During the hours or days of negative trends when symptoms worsen, one feels as if there is a return back to square one, but it is usually just a matter of one step back after two steps forward. Many of us learned about homeostasis in school. We were taught that nature tries to keep things within certain margins of optimal functioning. True enough, but nature's way always comes in waves so that "homodynamics" is a better word for the modulation of living systems. Everything about living things has to do with the integration of rhythms that* *often demand that we wait and see before we can judge the true trend of a certain event or symptom, especially in the developing child.*

* * * *

Through Dr. Sidney Baker, Judy was able to spread the word about SCD to other parents, and we soon had a core group of "Dr. Moms" who communicated daily via email about the effects that SCD had on our kids. These dedicated moms are the best and most courageous people I know. If there has been anything at all positive about this horrible experience, it has been getting to know these magnificent women. Amanda and I would never have made it without them.

For Amanda, there hasn't been an overnight change, but she has made slow and steady progress. At six months into SCD we introduced a quarter-teaspoon of goat yogurt, and for the first time she initiated a game of peek-a-boo with my mother. My mother and I both cried that day. It was hard to believe this was the same little girl who had been trapped in her own world for so long.

A month after we began SCD, Judy told me about Rudi Verspoor of the Hahnemann Center in Canada. Rudi started treating Amanda with sequential homeopathy, and we saw huge improvements once we started addressing the horrifying litany of insults that Amanda had suffered in her short life: the vaccines, steroids, and antibiotics all prescribed by her pediatricians.

After over two years of SCD and homeopathy, Amanda has gone from a 6:1:2 (six children, one teacher, and two aides) ABA class to attending a typical kindergarten with a shadow at our local elementary school. All on her own she goes to ballet class once a week, and she has just started Daisies, a junior Girl Scout troop with typical peers. She is still delayed in her expressive language and in her social skills, but I hope that one day she will be able to catch up. Every day she says something funny or smart, and I hug my daughter and give a prayer of thanks to Elaine Gottschall who helped make this miracle possible.

4. Anton's Story (from Russia), by Marina Solodovnikova

First of all, I want to say that I'm very much pro-SCD. I am absolutely sure that it is a very good diet and if I had a bit more will power I would be doing it myself too. Why didn't I come across it when I was 30, not 40+?

Secondly, I don't find it too difficult any more. But the thing is, even prior to SCD I didn't let Anton eat any processed food (even juice had always been freshly squeezed at home), so cooking had always been very time-consuming for me. The only additional thing is baking. So, I think the transition for me was easier than for most mums. It's more difficult for me though in the respect that in the cold season I have very limited access to vegetables like cauliflower, marrow, broccoli, and such like, so I'm basically down to cabbage, carrots, and red beets. I have cucumbers and tomatoes of course, but they are not filling enough. My other problem is that I've got no car, and buying *loads* more (compared to a regular diet) vegetables and fruit is not an easy task. However, it is certainly worth it.

The real difficulty was getting over Anton's upsets about not eating things he used to like. However, we managed to get over it. Occasionally he would ask me: "Why can't I have a sweetie? Why are other children eating them?" But I know that now he has new favorite things, and getting a piece of a cream cake (nut flour sponge with butter+honey+vanilla cream), a bunch of grapes or a bowl of yogurt (with banana, honey, or honey-based jam) is very rewarding for him. For all school parties I buy grapes and sometimes make cakes. And now of course we have started making ice cream from yogurt, which is a great success!

The main benefit of SCD for us is that I know that my son eats well. I think that I manage to balance protein with carbohydrates, because he eats *loads* of fruit and vegetables every day. Prior to SCD he only liked bananas; now he loves most fruit. He eats apples, pears, and bananas every day, and grapes every day in summer, autumn, and occasionally in winter and spring. In summer also strawberries and other berries, whatever comes our way. He doesn't like melon, but occasionally will eat a piece. Cabbage, carrots, and onions—virtually every day—and beets four or five days a week. Marrow, cauliflower, or broccoli stewed or fried makes his supper in summer and autumn. I often use eggs or cheese (or both) on vegetables to make them more filling. Mushrooms occasionally.

I use almond flour a lot. I make a sponge loaf, and Anton has a piece for breakfast (after an omelet), and I pack it with a banana for his snack at school. Also I make puddings with it: banana, carrot, or pumpkin, which is: eggs, flour, and grated carrot, pumpkin (with a bit of honey), or mashed banana mixed together and baked in the oven. Anton *loves* it as much as pancakes.

Yogurt—it is a *great* hit for us. However, I don't see anything good or bad that I could link to yogurt. Obsessive-compulsive stuff is very bad, but it had been bad before I introduced it. Many moms credit yogurt with significant improvements in social skills, but I haven't noticed anything in this respect, either. Anton has a big bowlful of yogurt every day now, which makes us both very happy. I buy milk from a woman who keeps her own cows; the milk is very fatty and the yogurt is really creamy, thick, and filling. Anton has put on a bit of weight since he started eating it.

Since Anton started SCD we have seen two major improvements: 1) Significant decrease in aggressive behaviors. Anton used to hit me very, very hard when he was angry with me for some reason. At the end of July we started doing SCD and large doses of oils, and ever since he hasn't hit me once. 2) Regular BMs. Constipation has been a very bad problem ever since Anton's birth. In March 2002 he had a prolapse (that is, the entire wall of the rectum is pushed out through the anus) after he hadn't had a BM for three or four days. It was a very frightening experience for Anton and for all of the family. It is a lot better now, also due to the oils and SCD. I've noticed that when we miss flax seed oil for a few days Anton constipates again. So, I think that it plays a great role in his BMs. However, I am sure that an enormous amount of fruit also does its good work. As quite a few moms claim that SCD helped a lot with aggressive behavior, I tend to think that it might be a combination of the two factors (SCD and flax seed oil) that is at work here.

5. Max's Story

I looked through the glass window and saw Max's hand raised eagerly to answer every question during the play last week at the children's museum. I wanted to shout, "YES!" but refrained since the teacher and other moms on the school trip knew nothing of Max's past. You see, it wasn't always like this.

Max was born in late October 1999. He was the perfect infant and even lifted his head in the hospital, so it wasn't a surprise that he could throw a ball across the room before he could walk. He was a good baby, the kind other people would be envious of. By a year, he was so easy to take care of, it was like he wasn't even there most of the time. I would later learn that was because he literally *wasn't* "there" most of the time.

By 18 months, Max was waking up screaming in the middle of the night with stomach pains. I remember him doing a weird twisting thing with his hands one night, but at the time I chose not to think about it. However, the strange obsessions, such as opening and closing doors and playing for hours with magnetic letters, were undeniable. The stomach pains would continue, and coincide with his numerous ear infections and doses of antibiotics, and were accompanied by chronic yellow-green, mushy stools. And after almost a year of trying to teach him his body parts, he could only identify his head. When these oddities were brought up to our pediatrician, he seemed unconcerned except for the obvious gastrointestinal symptoms. This was followed by a string of doctors with no answers.

Right before his second birthday our worst fears were realized, and Max was diagnosed with a pervasive developmental disorder with mild autistic tendencies. We were told that he might never speak and to get as much therapy for him as possible. His neurologist said it was a grey area because he was really too young to diagnose. However, six months later there was no mistaking that Max was truly autistic, and we were left devastated and with few answers.

The succeeding months were filled with frantic searches for answers without a clue as to where to begin. Then, as luck would have it, my mother came across a copy of *Unraveling the Mystery of Autism* by Karyn Seroussi. The story of her young son overcoming autism with dietary intervention was riveting. I stayed up all night reading her book, and within a day Max was gluten- and casein-free. Within a few days, Max could identify six body parts, and—before our very eyes—started to "wake up." It was a miracle. However, another ear infection and antibiotic wiped out much of this progress, and during this time I was called to pick him up from his special education program for diarrhea. He also seemed to have trouble walking and keeping his balance. Although this eased up after the antibiotics were finished, balance would continue to be a problem for a long time. Eventually Max got back on his feet but didn't rebound as quickly as we had hoped. It was around this time that my father saw an advertisement for a conference at which Karyn Seroussi and Dr. Sidney Baker were presenting. We eagerly attended, and there we met Dr. Baker who, to our great fortune, agreed to treat Max.

Under Dr. Baker's care, Max made incredible progress and things were moving along well. Max had left his ABA program and was moved to an integrated class. We continued on the GFCF diet but found that it still didn't seem to be giving him the jump he needed. We started experimenting by pulling out soy, corn, potatoes, and many other starches. As we removed more and more, Max started showing obvious improvements. We finally settled on rice being the grain of choice. Over time, Max craved rice products so badly that he was rarely eating something that didn't contain rice. He was happy to eat rice bread, rice waffles, rice crackers, rice cakes, and rice pasta all day. It didn't seem right, but what would he eat if we pulled the rice? What also didn't seem right was his continued unformed yellow stools, but I had no idea what to do. Then one day while on an Internet chat group, I saw a post for a new diet called the Specific Carbohydrate Diet.

Reports stated that SCD could be a very important diet; what struck me was that it didn't contain rice. I was scared to try a new diet but relieved to finally find a potential non-rice alternative diet for Max. I quickly got a copy of Elaine's book *Breaking the Vicious Cycle*, and once again overhauled Max's diet. For us the change was not drastic since the only non-SCD food that Max was eating was rice. I sometimes wonder if being so close to SCD while on GFCF was one of the reasons for Max's incredibly quick rate of improvement during the ensuing year and a half. I joined another chat group for children starting SCD in October 2003 and we were on our way. I figured that the diet might help a bit but I was not at all prepared for what followed:

This was my first post at almost three weeks on SCD when the improvements were becoming obvious:

> *Hi List,*
>
> *Just wanted to give you an update on my almost-four-year-old. We were GFCF for one and a half years with good results. Then I took away potatoes and corn about a year ago with even better results. The only illegal was rice, but now I can see what that was doing to him.*
>
> *Now, we are seeing great language improvements. Today he came up to me with something broken and said, "I can't fix it." The other night while crying, when asked why he was crying he said, "Want to go down. Want to see mommy." He's also using words that are not as concrete, like "I," "it" and "something." In the supermarket today, he looked at the number of the aisle and said, "It's number three" instead of just*

"Three." For him, these slight differences make his speech sound so much better. His therapist, who hasn't seen him since pre-SCD, said that his voice sounded more natural and he was just "quicker" all around. The best treat of all is that he's just coming up to me for no apparent reason and is saying, "Mommy!" He says it in a way someone would say hi. It's just so sweet.

Three weeks ago, he wouldn't touch any vegetables. Now he is eating squash fries, broccoli fries, and beet chips (all homemade). I was so happy when he ate his hamburger, broccoli fries, and pears for dinner.

Only one week later I wrote:

Hi list,

We are currently at four weeks SCD (Max was four years old yesterday), and here is the latest. We are continuing to see language improvements that are really great and obvious. This morning, we went outside and he said, "It's cold out." Also he asked, "Where are markers?" using "are" for the first time. School reports much better improvements in eye contact with other children. This was always harder for him than looking at adults. He spends half the day with NT kids in an integrated class and just loves being with them. OK, this is the good!

Max had his first formed stool and I was proud to report it!

At this time, a group of moms who are friends, whose children were also on SCD and who were also pursuing DAN! treatments, formed a little private support chat group called "Dr. Moms," and my opportunities for communicating with other moms continued. Soon after, these wonderful women would become some of my dearest friends.

By five months on the diet, I was telling the Dr. Moms about Max's now-dramatic improvements:

...Yesterday Max picked up my cell phone and said, "Hello," and then he carried on a conversation and said, "Goodbye." I asked him who he was talking to and he said, "Daddy." This is especially emotional for me since one of the last pre-ASD typical behaviors he had at around 11 months was picking up the toy phone and saying, "Hewow." It's as if he's picking up where he left off.

We had his IEP meeting and he is being recommended to go into the 15-1-2 special education kindergarten. It is not an ASD class and he will have mainstreaming opportunities. The district was amazed and even one of the pediatricians we saw today couldn't believe the difference from a few months ago.

And at six months:

[We] are getting loads of new spontaneous language. His play is getting better slowly. I saw him take his cars and put a traffic light in the middle of the scene—a small move but at least in the right direction. The other day at school a little boy said, "I'm going to build a car," and he said, "I'm going to build a house." This was huge for him to answer another child. He is much better with adults. It's hard for me to know exactly what is accounting for the big leap recently... but for sure, the diet has been the backbone for all the other treatments...

Because of the regressions that occurred, that first year was definitely the hardest, but it was also the most exciting in terms of Max's improvements. He has been on SCD for two and a half years now with a few more regressions but with truly unbelievable progress in terms of both his health (and bowels) and the elimination of all his autistic symptoms.

Without a doubt, SCD has truly been the foundation of all this progress, allowing other therapies to work even better. My son now attends a typical kindergarten class independently and only gets services for speech and OT. Max is reading, writing, playing with his friends, fighting with his sister, and doing most things a typical six-year-old does. There are still delays and he is socially immature but he's all there, well on his way toward his future, and succeeding at it all without anyone knowing all he's been through. Without SCD, this would not be possible.

Thank you Elaine, for making it possible for others to share in your success, and for helping to give me my son back!

* * * *

Dr. Baker: *Intelligence and maturation proceed in a developing child at rates that are not always tightly linked with chronological age. This is true in normal children, and the disparate rate of growth of intelligence and acquisition* *of maturity is even more marked in many very intelligent children.*

When I was Director of the Gesell Institute in New Haven, Connecticut, I had the privilege of meeting members of our national lecture staff who consulted for school systems around the United States, helping educators learn skills needed for assessing developmental maturity. When visiting schools, I heard from veteran teachers who were skeptical of educational consultants but who were effusive about our staff. "In my 20 years of teaching, I never have had such an easy time teaching as I have had after my children were grouped according to their maturity—as opposed to IQ or chronological age," was the message I heard from teachers. Parents who were reluctant to have their bright child "stay back" were relieved when he became happy to go to school and experienced success after being placed according to his maturity.

Maturation cannot be rushed, and upon its pace depend many learning skills. These may be very hard to master until a level of maturity is achieved when they suddenly become a snap. We do not insist that a four-year-old learn to ride a two-wheeler, nor do we think that a girl is less intelligent if her first period comes later than it does for the other girls. Maturation has its own pace. Of all our jobs as parents, the most important one is helping our children become self-confident. Achievement of self-confidence depends on timing. That is, if you try to get a four-year-old to learn to ride a two-wheeler, he will experience failure. If you let him learn at age six, he will experience success. If you are afraid to have him try until he has the maturity typical of eight-year-olds because you worry that he will crash and break a collar bone, he will feel your lack of confidence. More reason, then, to understand how to gauge you child's maturity and to be particularly aware that very bright babies seem to be at higher risk for the factors that induce autism. They may exhibit the persistent developmental immaturity that characterizes bright neurotypical children. We who are watching the details of our children's "behaviors" benefit from keeping the difficulties of the bright, immature child in mind as we assess their hyperactivity, problems with attention, and difficulties with socialization. A component of these problems may be due to simply not being ready, and therapies intended to remediate them may succeed only when children have been given the gift of time.

* * * *

6. Aidan's Story, by Heather Flaherty, R.N.

"Fifteen more minutes! You can do it, Aidan... you can do it!"

Now, if I can just get dinner done before Robin finishes running this play date for him, I am golden. I'm finding it hard to swallow right now... I'm going to stop watching. Real Moms don't watch every second of their kids' play dates. Better busy myself making dinner before that mom comes back to pick up her child. God, I hope he wants to come back. Let's see... I'll do the usual tonight, some gluten-free french fries, because it makes him so happy. Happy—that's something less and less frequently experienced these days. At least I feel normal making these french fries. Besides, I just need him to eat without a struggle tonight. I need a break from the tantrums.

"Aidan, say goodbye," "Aidan, wave," "Aidan, what do you say when a friend leaves?" "Aidan, do you want him to come back?" "You need to use words, Aidan."

I quickly scan to see the mother's face as she is scooping up her son. The look. The look that says, "I can't believe that you treat your son like a dolphin at Sea World. I hope you didn't talk to my son like that."

"Thank you."

"We will have to do this again. Your son was so helpful teaching Aidan how to go up and down the slide."

"Yes, maybe again sometime."

"OK, he doesn't want to stay for dinner? It is french fries... OK, thanks again for coming."

"Mommy, french fries?"

"Yes, honey, you earned it!"

And then Robin, Aidan's therapist, breaks the news to me.

"Heather, I just wanted to tell you that when Aidan was going up the slide he had yellow liquid smear the slide and it's on his pants."

"Oh, I'm sorry! It's this medicine for his diarrhea and belly pain. It is bright yellow and stains. I'm sorry you had to clean it. I was watching. Did he do OK?"

"It's still the same. He needs a lot of prompting and still seems spaced out and disconnected. Maybe we should put a hold on the typical kids coming over. It is still too hard for him. He needs more one-to-one."

"No, please Robin. It gives me hope. He needs a friend. It is normal to have play dates at his age."

I feel the tears in my throat. Yup, I can do it... push it down, down, down.

"Well, we will talk about it again. Go help him. He's in the bathroom again. See you tomorrow. I'll bring new flashcards."

"Hi, honey. How is your belly?"

"New undies! New undies! New undies!"

"Hang on, Aidan. Let's clean this up and off you go to the counter. If you can just hang on while I clean this up you can have your french fries."

Dinner was faster tonight. No vomiting. Boy, this GFCF diet isn't so bad. A lot of baking, but I can do it. I'll save the GFCF cupcakes for feeding therapy tomorrow. Supplements and we are done. I'll get my walk in tonight. Dad can do the bath.

"Daddy!"

"Hi, Aidan."

I am out of here. I need to walk and get a break. Everything is done.

"Can you just play with him and give him a bath?"

"Sure thing. And try to smile."

"Yeah."

I am missing something. Walk faster. I am. I know it. He has two-word sentences. At least he's talking again. We have a gastroenterologist. We see allergists, we see immunologists, we see everybody. Why isn't he getting any better? The air feels good. I just need to keep thinking. Maybe I will start that antifungal tomorrow.

Oh no!!! The lights are still on. Not again. I can't take this! I am going insane. Maybe I can just sit here and wait. Brendan can do it… he can take care of it. I'll just sit here on the front steps and they won't even know I'm back.

"HEATHER!!! You had better…"

SCREAM

"… come…"

SCREAM

"… up!"

SCREAM

"He's vomiting again and he feels really hot!"

I can do it. Up the stairs. My baby needs me. There he is, white as a ghost, staring at me with those eyes that were once bright blue, now gray, almost black, with circles the size of the rings of Saturn under his eyes, vomit on his onesie.

"What did you feed him?! Is it those french fries again? Did he have a play date? Maybe he caught something again. You need to call that company, I think there is something in those fries... No more play dates! He has no immune system. Heather, come on."

Can't I just go for a walk? Did you make him laugh too hard? He ate so nicely tonight.

WHY?

So there I sit, holding my boy, telling him it's OK, while he holds his ever-so-swollen belly and my husband cleans up the vomit and gets the Tylenol.

"I'll take him back to the pediatrician tomorrow. They'll tell me it's just another virus. The immunologist wants to start IV immunoglobulin treatments, did I tell you that?"

"What is that?"

"Never mind."

I am missing something.

Aidan is asleep now, in my arms.

Brendan says, "Can you put him to bed, please?"

"Oh, I'm sorry. I just can't stop thinking and trying to..."

"Just put him to bed."

The sadness in my husband's voice is raw, almost sharp.

Off I go to the bed, where we all sleep together. "Thank God," I think, as I put my ear over Aidan's belly. "Thank God we have this closeness at night. No therapists telling me what to do with you. Just you and me and Daddy." He lets me hold him at night. I have my usual private talk with his belly, begging, begging it to tell me what it needs to heal. "I don't know how you got to this. Please, give me a sign of hope. What am I missing?"

That was our private hell. No one but immediate family knew this hell. It went on for two years, along with anaphylaxing to different foods, the wet leaves during the autumn, touching a Christmas tree... We were down to rotating a small list of foods. We carried Aidan's EpiPen (a shot full of adrenaline for severe allergic reactions) wherever we went. Anaphylaxis: the closing of his throat so that he couldn't breathe, followed by shock, loss of consciousness, and then near-death...

He was so thin and yet so bloated. For us, sailing in "calm" waters meant avoiding the hospital for a week, avoiding a feeding tube and other extreme measures.

"Mrs. Flaherty, you are amazing. I don't know how you keep him alive!"

Oh, how I hated that line. That nervous, uncomfortable scratch of the forehead that said, "I have no idea what to do with your child."

That is how we lived, in and out of Boston Children's Hospital. Asthma attacks, anaphylaxis, IV hydration, you name it. It would be a miracle if Aidan saw four years of age. We just couldn't keep our child healthy. He was three now. It would be time to transition to school soon, but how? Every other week he was on a home nebulizer system, missing hour upon hour of ABA. When he was in the hospital, I would flip flashcards, bring lacing cards and shape puzzles, for fear we were falling further and further behind. I was told Floortime could be done anywhere. We tried. We just kept trying. It was all we could do.

Time to meet the school district. Time to transition. We walked into the school saying nothing to each other, Brendan and I. We stared at what seemed like millions of children, going here and there and everywhere, coughing, sneezing... the smell of mold. We live in a historic port city. Beautiful, but old, schools.

"There is no way he will be able to breathe here," we told the director. "Thank you, but this won't work."

I could feel the heat rising in my face. I knew the blotches would come soon on my neck.

"What do you mean, Mrs. Flaherty?"

"Excuse me a moment and I can show you."

Off to the car I ran to get my five overstuffed binders of labs, hospitalizations, all beautifully color-coded. I was ready. They can't force me to put my son in this school. He'll die.

But he needs to go to school. He needs to be with other children.

My nightly private walks in the dark. Think. There has to be a way. I thought about the children I took care of, as a bone marrow transplant nurse, and how immune-compromised they were. There was a lot of help for them from companies and organizations. It can't hurt to ask, I thought.

The next day I called construction companies, Lowe's, and Home Depot. I wrote grants and finally Home Depot responded. A wonderful group of men came to my house and with my husband and some neighbors, built a schoolroom in our basement for Aidan that looked like a small classroom. Totally environmentally controlled. We hired a teacher. But Aidan was so alone, so isolated, so sad. He needed a role model or two. He needed friends.

I made flyers: "Looking for a healthy child to come to home school program two hours per week. Guaranteed fun. Mother a nurse and there will be a certified teacher."

We were very lucky. Friends poured in their support and I had one child for each day of the week. Still, Aidan missed weeks at a time as he went in and out of the hospital, and his PDD behaviors remained. He still hit, bit, smacked… and he was still in pain.

While sitting at a conference and watching a slide presentation of a little boy who looked just like my Aidan, I found the road to healing. I followed that presenter, Dr. Sidney Baker, into the men's room, begging for just five minutes of his time. Those five minutes turned my son's life around. Before that moment, I had almost given up hope.

Antifungals, secretin, BayGam, supplements, urine tests, stool tests. We watched and monitored, changed antifungals. Manipulated his supplements. He was getting better after round upon round of earth-shaking die-off of yeast. Aidan was connecting. He was engaging.

And I had found "game meats."

At this point, Aidan's list of severe food allergies was hundreds of items long. I needed to find things foreign to his immune system, which I could rotate. My husband was sent on a trip to purchase bear, turtle, lion, and alligator meats. I researched what these animals ate, cross-checked to make sure that Aidan was not allergic to anything in the animals' diets….

But Aidan was still getting rice pasta and french fries.

Another trip to Dr. Baker's. I was so excited to tell him of my new idea, to rotate game meats. He looked at me, pressed his lips together, and began telling me of his learning about a diet that seemed very promising. I remember thinking, "Oh no! He can't be! He can't be telling me to take even more away! Please, don't complicate this even more. And this is you, Dr. Baker—the one who throws me no curve balls!"

To him I said, "No WAY! There are nuts in that diet! I have looked into it and it is impossible! Remember, this is Aidan. He anaphylaxes with eggs, nuts…."

I quickly changed the subject. I can still see him reaching up to his shelf for that book….

But luckily, Dr. Baker didn't stop there. He asked another mom to call me. I barely knew her, having only met her briefly once before. He knew it would take a mother describing, with great force, how well her son was doing on SCD to get me to try this. She called on Aidan's birthday. I was busy cleaning up the GFCF cupcakes and present wrapping from the floor. I blocked out a bit.... After all, it was nice having a cupcake for your child on his birthday.

But then this mom said, "Yes, well, it may be nice for you, but what about him? This could really help, Heather. This could be it."

She knew I was beaten, tired, and scared. Aidan was still autistic. Better, yes, yet he was still soooooooooo sick.

"What do you have to lose?"

By the time she told me her son was out of his ABA classroom, I had two pantry shelves bare. Bag after bag of Miss Roben's foods went flying into the garbage. That is how I do things: cold turkey. No room for going back, no way to half do it. No games to be played. No dabbling with the diet. I forced myself to do it.

BANG! SLAM! SCREAM! YELL!

"I want RICE! I want RICE!!!!"

"You can't have it, Aidan. It's hurting your belly."

"I WANT RICE!!!!"

Later that day I decided to lock myself in the bathroom while Aidan's therapist worked with him—as he screamed for rice. I read *Breaking the Vicious Cycle* for a second time. Soon I had a reading rack installed in the bathroom... it wasn't such a bad place to hide out.

One month later my son had his first formed stool.

I had friends on the Internet now. I had my game meats to rotate, and three vegetables and three fruits. Aidan was living on this three times a day. But it didn't matter: he was talking in four- and five-word sentences. His behavior was better. He was in less pain.

"I can't believe that you are only going to give him that," someone would say. "Turtle meatballs and carrots for breakfast?! That is insane!"

Insane it might be to some. But we were staying out of the hospital. Aidan wasn't vomiting anymore. He was getting better.

After a year on SCD, Aidan was able to attend a typical preschool program with an aide. His immune system was so much stronger. He still ate his limited repertoire of foods... but it didn't matter because he was healing by the day. The therapy was getting in, the shades were lifting and the windows opening.

He was bored of his food so I had to become very creative, which isn't natural for me. Pear slices became the wings of an airplane on a stick, with the blueberries as the head of the pilot. I rolled and shaped ground organic veal into sausages, with hidden carrot juice inside.

It is a lot of work. I don't deny that for a second. But stop and think about how we run from physician to physician for answers. Therapists tell us what to do. Ads on TV tell us what to feed our kids, what makes them happy and what is "normal." Doing this diet makes me feel like a real mother—doing SCD started the healing of my severely sick and autistic child. I cooked, peeled, and chopped. I designed his menu with five meat choices and three fruits and three vegetables. There are so many recipes that I can't use on this diet. But doing SCD with Aidan put me back in charge. I am back in control.

Every day I am doing something that makes him better.

Sure, the french fries make us feel great and, for a split second, they make our kids happy. We want normal so badly. We are tired. We have other children. We need easy.

But healing isn't easy. It takes work. This is my chance, I firmly believe, to hold the reins again as a mother.

So stop for a moment and think about your views on food. Why is it easier to continue what you are doing? Do the GFCF foods make you feel at least like you can give those so-called treats? Is it that your child has so many allergies that SCD seems impossible? Once you identify why you are hesitating, and are honest with yourself, you will see—as I did—that we *can* do it. There are gut linings that need a break. They need to heal.

Our children cannot live on antifungals forever.

We are now two years on SCD. Aidan is in a typical classroom at a private school with an aide to make sure he doesn't come into contact with any food he is highly allergic to. (Yes, she does some mild redirection academically.) But Aidan is no longer autistic. He isn't in pain. He is alive, getting healthy—and he is full of love.

* * * *

Judy's comments: This past summer, with Aidan so healed, Heather and her family were able to come for a visit to New York. Our two families spent the day together at an adventure park. We had lunch at my parents' house first, where Aidan spent some time discussing Egyptian artifacts with his dad, me, and my father, explaining to us what a sarcophagus was. My father leaned over to me and whispered, "This child was autistic?"

Yes, Dad. He was.

In two years, Aidan went from being just one step above a "bubble boy" to going onto the haunted house ride with me, the helicopters with my then eight-year-old son...

I talked to him on the phone a few nights ago. "Aidan, are you going to come to visit me again soon?" "Yes!" "Should we go to that park again and go on more rides?" "Yes, but I don't want to go into the haunted house again!"

* * * *

7. Eric's Story, by Sharie Ypsilanti

My son, Eric, was diagnosed with PDD in December 1995, after completing extensive testing and ruling out a hearing loss at about 18 months of age. This diagnosis was later confirmed, and he was called autistic by a second pediatric neurologist in January 1997, when he was 30 months

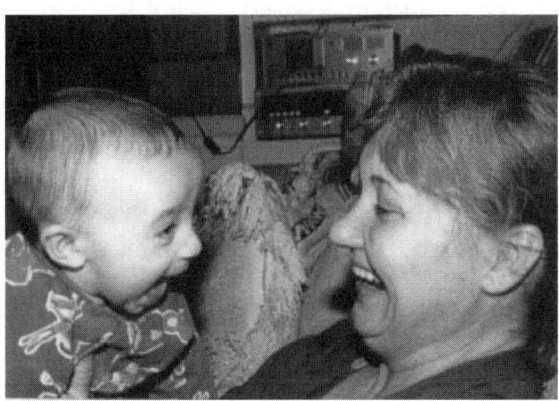

old. Later, in September 1998, a third doctor who specialized in genetics diagnosed Eric with pervasive developmental delay with autistic features after ruling out all known genetic syndromes. All of the testing completed by these doctors came back negative or normal.

My pregnancy with Eric was generally uneventful, except that I received a flu shot about two weeks after conceiving, I was sick twice during the second trimester, and once I received an antibiotic. Eric appeared completely normal for at least the first eight to nine months of his life. He was very irritable on regular formula, however, and had to be changed to soy formula while still in the hospital. He was diagnosed with chicken pox at four months, and it seemed like a mild case. When Eric was about almost three months old he started having frequent upper respiratory infections and was treated almost every time with antibiotics by the pediatric group. He was sick almost all the time, and then started getting diarrhea. He also had difficulty maintaining weight gain. The pediatrician recommended a low dose of antibiotics as a prophylactic measure, but we did not think it was a good idea and refused.

Eric's behavioral change was gradual and not immediately noticed. Looking back, his skills and growth seemed to plateau at about nine months of age. We were not overly concerned since Eric's older brother was a slow starter, but then progressed normally. When he was 14 months old, Eric slept through a fire alarm and then we started to notice other unusual behavior. He was generally very quiet and did not babble much. He had poor eye contact and did not respond any more to his name or even loud noises. He did not interact with others like he used to and no longer played with toys. He was frequently sick and did not sleep well at night. He cried a lot and kicked his legs. He was content to sit for long periods of time and stare at his fingers, and did not attempt to explore his environment except by excessive mouthing of objects.

Our pediatrician referred us to Blythedale Children's Hospital for an audiological evaluation in August of 1995. The evaluator told us that Eric exhibited selective hearing during the exam, and that was the first time the word autism was used. Eric was 14 months old. We were then sent to a specialist and went through a number of tests that all came back normal. What was not normal was Eric's response to medications that were supposed to put him to sleep for the MRI and EEG. They had the opposite effect and he became hyperactive. Those tests had to be rescheduled many times before he finally fell asleep. Also, he continued to have diarrhea and was especially sick with upper respiratory infections during the winter. Eric was also evaluated by Cardinal McCloskey Services for the Early Intervention Program and was found to be significantly delayed across all areas of development. He was functioning cognitively at an eight- to nine-month level, and his social and communication skills were at a five- to six-month level. He started receiving services (speech, PT, OT, and special education) at about 16 months of age at a center-based program. He had no separation anxiety at all and hardly seemed to recognize us.

When Eric was 21 months old, he was still not standing or bearing weight on his feet, and his muscle tone had deteriorated. He was not able to sit up well. We took him to a physiatrist who prescribed solid ankle-foot orthotics and a prone stander. Then we took him for an auditory brainstem evaluation later that month, which concluded that he had abnormal middle-ear functioning in the left ear. This was not surprising since he continued to have frequent upper respiratory infections.

When Eric was two years old, I read a book by Doris Rapp, *Is This Your Child's World?*, which discussed food allergies. I noticed Eric had the following symptoms of food allergies: chronic sinus infection, excessive perspiration and drooling, pale face with red blotches on cheeks, watery eyes, and sleep problems. I spoke to the pediatrician and she agreed to do a blood test for milk allergies; it came back positive. He was changed to a soy formula and he stood up independently two weeks later. The pediatrician referred us to an allergist who did skin testing and all the testing came back negative, even for milk. Our HMO did not approve any further testing for allergies. Then when Eric was two and a half years old, the winter of 1996, he started having major difficulties at night. He was unable to sleep very long, cried, screamed and needed constant comforting, and he started to demonstrate self-abusive behaviors. He would hit his ears and face until he bled. He had to be swaddled in a quilt in a dark room and rocked around the clock. In January of 1997, we took him to yet another doctor who told us that she felt Eric was autistic, had microscopic brain damage that did not show up on the MRI, and would most likely never walk. He was still chronically congested, and had nasal discharge, diarrhea, fevers, and tantrums.

Finally, in March of 1997 when he was about 33 months old, Eric started walking. In June of that year, when Eric was turning three, I made an appointment with an allergist and immunologist. He diagnosed Eric as having an immune dysfunction, with allergies to several foods (dairy, soy, nuts, gluten, and eggs). He recommended a change in his diet and IVIG therapy. We changed Eric's diet in August and took him off gluten and all allergens, but were unable to start IVIG therapy until January of 1998 when we changed insurance companies. We did see an improvement right away with the diet. Eric slept better, was happier, and was making some progress in school until December. At that point, he got swollen glands behind his ears, was very pale, threw tantrums, and hit his ears until they bled. In January of 1998, Eric started receiving 10 grams of intravenous gamma globulin (Gamma Guard) every three weeks. This continued until May of 2002. There was significant improvement on the IVIG therapy. Eric got only one or two upper respiratory infections a year and was usually able to recover without antibiotics. He grew, gained weight, and his muscle tone improved. He learned to jump, run, and kick a ball (although awkwardly). He was more energetic, attentive, and responsive. His self-abusive behavior decreased dramatically. He continued to be extremely hyperactive, however, and severely autistic. He required a one-to-one aide in school because of severe pica.

When Eric was five years old he was unable to sit in a chair for more than a couple of minutes. We made the decision to medicate him for hyperactivity. We took him to a developmental pediatrician who prescribed Prozac. Eric had a manic reaction to the Prozac and so the doctor decided to raise his dose. Eric went totally out of control and was violently self-abusive. We took Eric back to one of our doctors who took him off Prozac and prescribed Clonidine in the AM and PM. Eric calmed down, and a month later was also prescribed Risperdal. Eric did relatively well for a while, but then sometime in the fall of 2000, I let the immunologist convince me to take him off Nystatin. In December, Eric started having issues with food. Whenever it was time to eat he would start crying. The self-abusive behavior increased, and he became unmanageable at times. It would come and go. He had a lot of gas and belched a lot. We at first assumed it was behavioral and tried increasing medications and behavioral interventions.

We went on vacation in June of 2001 and Eric became abusive toward others for the first time. He didn't want to eat much, was inconsolable, and could not sleep. When we returned, we went to a new doctor, who immediately thought it might be his stomach and ordered several GI tests and put him back on Nystatin. The *H. pylori* test came back positive and Eric was put on Biaxin and Amoxicillin for that, along with Prilosec. He was still having great difficulty though, and was hospitalized at Westchester County Medical Center for several days. He was found to be constipated and had a fever prior to admission and he was put on vancomycin (an intestinal antibiotic) IV for four days and treated for constipation. Eric was like a different child. This was a major clue as to what was wrong with Eric, but at that time, we really didn't understand.

Eric was referred to a gastroenterologist for an endoscopy and had one at Mt. Sinai. The doctor found some mild inflammation in the esophagus and concluded that Eric had some mild pain that was exaggerated by his personality. By September of 2001, Eric's behavior was out of control again and I called our new immunologist, who referred us to a second pediatric gastroenterologist.

Our new gastroenterologist did another endoscopy and also a colonoscopy and found swollen lymph nodes in Eric's colon, but no other inflammation. He concluded that the main problem was constipation and recommended mineral oil in the evenings. Eric seemed to improve after the colonoscopy, but not for long. By the end of November he had pulled out all the hair on top of his head and was head-banging.

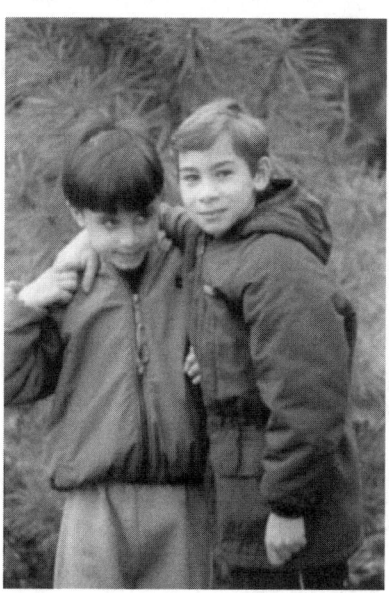

Eric and his big brother, Evan (look closely at the top of Eric's head— you can see the spot where he'd pulled out the first clump of hair)

At that point, we had to get a helmet for Eric. He was always gassy, belching, spitting up, and very unhappy. He was in constant pain. Our immunologist prescribed Prevacid, which did help somewhat. He also told me to increase the mineral oil and the Nystatin, and he started giving Eric secretin infusions every four to five weeks. When Eric would have a really bad episode, the doctor would give him a cortisone shot. Eric's school was having difficulty controlling him and recommended residential placement. He had to leave his school in January of 2002 and go to a special school with a higher staff ratio and more nursing care for the profoundly retarded. Unfortunately, Eric continued to have severe GI problems, which impacted upon his progress and behavior. Again, we went back to the gastroenterologist. We tried Azulfidine, Prednisone, chelation therapy, and a two-month trial of vancomycin. The biggest improvement occurred during the two times he was on vancomycin and the short-term prednisone therapy. But these measures never seemed to last and before we knew it, Eric was in crisis again.

The gastroenterologist saw Eric in his office in August of 2003. Eric was stooped over in a posture with his heel in his anus, screaming, crying, and banging his head on the floor. If anyone came near him he would pull at their hair, clothes, or jewelry. If we attempted to hold him he hit us with his head. This had been going on since early July, two to five times a day. It had been getting worse and he was obviously in extreme pain. The gastroenterologist put him on a clear liquid diet for the next 48 hours. We gave Eric soda on the way home and we were surprised there were no complaints about missing dinner. He seemed calmer and slept 12 hours that night, which was highly unusual. Overall, Eric seemed happier on the liquid diet. He smiled more and did not scream so much. He still did have some pain, but the episodes were fewer, shorter, and did not seem as intense as before. He also slept for longer periods and seemed more relaxed. When I reported back to the doctor, he prescribed Modulen, an irritable bowel disease formula, for Eric to continue on until further notice. Eric's behavior certainly improved on this diet at first. Initially, his self-inflicted wounds healed and he did not pull at people as much as he used to. It was good to see him smile. However, he still had pain, especially in the morning. He did not seem to miss food as much as he missed chewing. He was chewing many things and swallowed newspaper, mail, and even his own diaper whenever he got the chance.

In September of 2003, the gastroenterologist did another endoscopy and colonoscopy on Eric. He was unable to do a complete colonoscopy due to extensive feces found in the ileal section of Eric's colon, even though he had prepped Eric the previous day. The doctor did find several ulcers in the duodenum and stool in the stomach and esophagus. Eric remained on the Modulen and was prescribed more Azulfidine and Miralax for the constipation. As the weeks passed, Eric's symptoms worsened and he was prescribed Prednisone, which Eric refused to take by mouth and had to get via weekly shots. His condition continued to deteriorate. A series of lab tests was performed in November. Eric was found to have a lead level of 30, so began a series of EDTA shots, which reduced his lead level to 15 by December. The source of the lead is our apartment in Bronxville, which had to be renovated by a lead removal-certified contractor.

But by January of 2004, Eric was crying most of the day and night, self-abusive and increasingly aggressive. One day, Eric's school called 911 to transport him to the nearest hospital, since I was unable to transport him myself because of his extreme behavior. Mt. Vernon Hospital gave him an abdominal x-ray and found about 10 screws and some other objects in his intestines. They were all clumped together in one area. He was transport-ed to Montefiore Children's Hospital. Eric was completely out of control for 26 hours before he fell asleep exhausted. He was in the hospital until a colonoscopy was done to break up the impaction and remove the objects from his colon. During that time he was placed on a clear liquid diet; he lost 10 pounds before the impaction moved to the large intestine through the ileal cecal valve. Our gastroenterologist correctly predicted that Eric would continue to have pain when the impaction was removed because he felt the pain was from a flare-up of Eric's colitis.

In February Eric was in crisis again and was once again prescribed 40mg of Prednisone, which we started the next day. Eric improved for four days, and then his self-abusive and aggressive behavior returned. He was given Tylenol with codeine and then Endocet for pain, but nothing seemed to help. It was only then that the doctor realized that Eric had gone into steroid psychosis (if you take large doses of steroids for too long, it can make you go crazy) and he lowered the Prednisone gradually. During this time I was in contact with Judy, and she convinced both our gastroenter-ologist and me to try the Specific Carbohydrate Diet. Since the doctor felt that he had done all he could with Eric, his next step would have be to hos-pitalize him, insert a feeding tube, and wire his jaw shut. I was adamantly against that, so Eric started the SCD on March 4, 2004.

The first six days on the diet were amazing. Eric did not have one episode of self-abuse or aggression. He ate and slept well and seemed happy. After that there was a marked regression, which continued through the end of March. He had a lot of gas, belching, and discomfort. However, he also began having regular BMs, and there was no sign of undigested food in his stool.

Eric was first seen by Dr. Sidney Baker in April of 2004. Sid prescribed vancomycin, gentamycin, and Sporanox. There was a good response to the genta/vanco combination: Eric was less constipated, less gassy, and generally happier. However, he continued to have problems with aggression and self-abuse the entire summer of 2004. He even broke his right elbow in a self-abusive rage. Sid prescribed BayGam in July, which seemed to help, but Eric continued to have difficulty. We started working with a new neurologist in June, because even the residential placement was refusing to accept Eric because of his aggression. The neurologist prescribed several psychotropic drugs and dosages before we finally found the right combination. Sid was also trying to stabilize Eric, and give him some relief. He sent Eric's blood to Dr. Jill James and got the thiol profiles. Eric needed glutathione and P5P/MCB/folinic AC/NAC shots. He had been getting the shots, but not enough and not with P5P. Eric started receiving these supplements in November and we noticed continued improvement.

On November 2, 2004, Eric was admitted to Ferncliff Manor, a residential placement for developmentally delayed children with medical conditions. It was a very difficult decision for us, but one that had to be made. Eric had not been safe with us for awhile. The pica caused Eric to eat any non-edible object he could get his hands on, and he had started walking out the front door both at our apartment and at our house on Shelter Island. Eric needed 24-hour one-to-one supervision, which we were unable to get. In addition, he needed a school that could handle his medical needs. In my mind, I was giving up and I thought Eric would have a lower standard of living than we could provide him. I felt trapped; I had no choices really, but the one thing I wanted to do was keep him close to home. Ferncliff is six miles from our apartment and across the street from where I work.

What we found at Ferncliff amazed us. Sid Baker is able to continue to manage Eric's medical care. The dietician and kitchen staff strictly follow the SCD. Eric has a one-to-one aide 24 hours a day. He is in one of the largest classes he's ever been in (12 kids) with various exceptionalities, and he loves school for the first time ever! He receives PT, OT, and speech services, and almost all his doctors come to him. He is still followed once a month by the neurologist who has stated that he has never before witnessed such a dramatic change in a child. Everyone asks me what I attribute the progress to. My answer is that Eric needed a doctor like Sid, who would spend hours talking and thinking about him; a doctor like our neurologist who would try every medication and combination; a diet like SCD that would help his GI system; and a place like Ferncliff, with a huge staff trained to work with and pay attention to a child like Eric.

Eric still has a long way to go. He is 11 years old and weighs just 64 pounds. He is still in diapers, but he does sit on the toilet now. He still wears a helmet sometimes. Because he is still nonverbal he sometimes gets frustrated with his inability to communicate. But I don't think Eric is in pain now—I think he has gotten used to using self-abusive behavior to express his feelings and demonstrate how strongly he feels about things. And

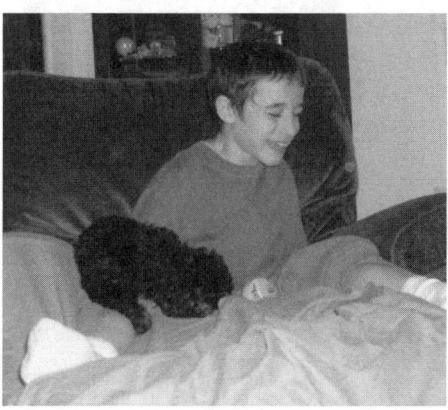

Eric with Winnie, his new puppy

I think he is also manipulative. He does occasionally have pain I'm sure, but I call to check up on him continually and he is perfectly happy. It's only when I go to see him that he will start banging his head on a wall, often as soon as he sees me! He has never been aggressive at Ferncliff... what does that tell you? At Ferncliff he's a perfect little angel! The pica has improved a lot, although there are certain things he definitely cannot pass up. He is able to wear regular clothes now because he doesn't try to eat his diaper anymore. I'm just trying to maintain Eric with what we have, which is a lot.

Since we started Eric on SCD, we have not had to rush to the hospital once or call a doctor in the middle of the night. Eric's health and behavior have stabilized. His receptive language and communication skills have increased. And now we both have a social life!

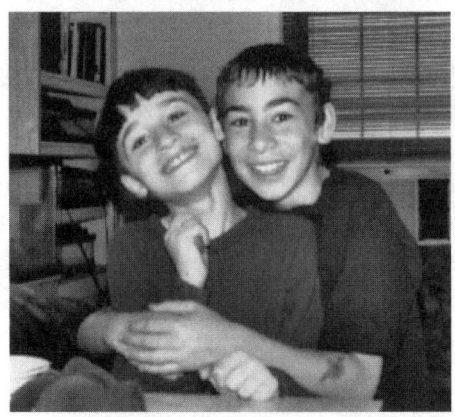

Eric and his big brother

* * * *

Judy's comments: About four months after I'd started Alex on SCD, around the time I started to see the first improvements, I volunteered to have Alex give blood for a study. He and I arrived at the lab to discover a scene of complete chaos. There were about 15 families, all with autistic children (who were all fasting, which made the children that much more insane), crammed into a tiny waiting room that was about 100 degrees. There weren't nearly enough chairs for all of us, so people were sitting on the floors. One kid was eating the plants while another was pulling over the water cooler. I turned to a mom waiting near the door and asked how long she'd been waiting. "About two hours now," she said, "but there are people who were here well before me."

Well, as you can imagine, my first reaction was to walk straight out; but then—thank goodness—I changed my mind. I figured I'd wait at least a little while because the line might start to move and I didn't want to give up my chance at getting the information from the lab test. Alex and I squeezed our way in and eventually found a seat and I started to chat with the woman next to me. Sharie told me that her son was in the car with her husband because he was so sick that she couldn't possibly bring him into a crowd like this. She then admired how well my son was doing! That was a first.

But then again, it was the first time I had met a parent of a child who was even sicker than Alex. When Sharie's husband finally brought in their little boy, Eric, for the blood draw, my insides clenched up. I just barely kept myself from bursting into tears on the spot. It is a moment I will never forget. Even today I can hardly bear the memory of my first look at Eric, wearing his helmet, his pants barely held on by a belt because he was so thin....

I can't write any more about it. Three years later and I am still crying now.

Sharie told me in detail how Eric was violently self-abusive, often very aggressive, and had terrible gastrointestinal symptoms. So of course, I launched into an impassioned speech about the glories of SCD and what it had done for us already. Sharie and I ended up having hours together in that horrible place, and there's not a day that goes by when I'm not thankful for every minute of it.

My new friend didn't say "I can't do it," or "It's too hard," or "All he wants to eat is crackers." In spite of everything she and her family were going through, a few months after we met she put Eric on SCD. Fourteen months or so after our meeting, she wrote the following to me:

> "I will always remember your persistence and help in getting us on the right track concerning SCD. I am here today to tell you that it's made all the difference in the world in terms of the quality of our lives.... Eric is doing great and has been truly stable for months now. He has no more pain and very little gas and has begun to gain weight—although he is still very thin. He is laughing again and has been very responsive.... Eric is on the road to good health and he is happy.... I realize how lucky we were to meet you that day in the lab. What if I hadn't spoken to you, or what if the lab had its act together and we had been in and out of there and never met?"

* * * *

8. Letters from Elaine's Files

A. Kevin continues to amaze us with his progress. We have had four "perfect," calm, happy days with unbelievable mental activity and progress.

This has never happened before. Not only are we thrilled, we are shocked, mystified. He wants to be constantly engaged in stimulating activities, is actually playing by himself and with his brother (as opposed to crying or screaming), and wants to learn, is inquisitive, goes to bed and sleeps, takes himself to the bathroom, etc.

Thanks to all of you and especially Elaine. You are all making this miracle happen.

B. We have been SCD for two months and loving every minute of it. The positive gains are so encouraging. Every day my children are getting better and better. My daughter, who has an autism diagnosis, is doing great. She is communicating more every day (for example, "Where have you been, Mom?"), and actually carrying on a conversation back and forth. I am thrilled. I made a promise to myself last year that I didn't care what I had to do, that I was going to heal my children if it is the last thing that I do. Elaine, you are a godsend, and we love you for caring about our children, and bringing them back to us. My daughter is functioning beautifully in typical first grade. She is making friends and socializing. She is even getting in trouble for talking in class. My son had dyspraxia of speech and severe sensory integration issues, but that is all in the past. He is now talking up a storm and is very active. He's not the same kid. And my two-year-old daughter, who is speech-delayed, is talking more and more every day. The magic bullet is proper nutrition that so many kids' bodies are starving for.

I feel like I am truly blessed and am having the life that I was supposed to have. My life was perfect after my daughter was born. She was so beautiful and innocent until she received the MMR at 13 months, and then our nightmare began. All of her language stopped and as time went on she was sinking into her own world. But now my beautiful little girl is coming back. I will keep everyone posted as progress is made.

C. Matthew went to see Dr. Bradstreet the other day, and what a tremendous change from our last visit, two months ago, pre-SCD. No more mad giggles and stimming, he sat there in his office just fine. Dr. B. was very pleased but not surprised (he apparently has been recommending SCD quite a bit) and simply said, okay, we found something that works, keep it up and we'll see you in three months.

And now for our progress report...

Matthew seems to be over his setback, it started after four weeks and it ended up lasting three weeks, and I am guessing it was due to a combo of allowing whole nuts and too much fruit. I have cut out the nuts and will be severely limiting the fruit, and probably using enzymes when he has fruit.

He of course has calmed down considerably and is no longer the constantly stimming, madly giggling boy he was a few months ago.

He is now *using* his PECS symbols in exactly the way his therapist wants him to—pulling them out of his notebook and bringing them to me. He used to rely on taking us by the hand and dragging us around the house, which he still does a little but not nearly as much. I have a hard time telling him no to anything when he is asking me so nicely!

Here is the *major* breakthrough—are you ready—he is GOING TO BED BY HIMSELF!!! Daddy takes him in the room (at 8:30!) and tells him good-night, go to sleep, and he STAYS IN THERE AND GOES TO SLEEP!!! Sorry for the all caps but this is major—we used to have to wait until he calmed down and passed out on the floor. He is getting heavier and I had images of me hoisting a twelve-year-old off the floor and into his bed! He has always needed someone to stay with him at least until he fell asleep, and at worst he wouldn't go to sleep and we would have to take him to bed with us once 10 or 11 came. Hurrah!

D. I thought I would send in a progress report that might help lurkers who are on the fence about the diet, although I realize we've been unusually blessed so far, even by SCD standards. We are just seeing marvelous improvements every day in every aspect of my son's being. He is going to be four in November. He's been on the diet for a week and yesterday we had three trophies (formed bowel movements)!!!!! Today, again, the first BM is perfectly normal looking. And I could bore you for hours with all the behavioral improvements—greater energy, much more verbal, incredible pretend play. Yesterday this speech therapist brought over Fisher Price people and furniture and he made a little bathroom, bringing the toilet, bath, and sink together. Then he had the doll wash her hands and take a bath, talking appropriately all the while, with no prompting and no models. This is a child who, a month ago, only had enough pretend play to make a little noise when pushing a car, or make an animal pretend to eat for a moment or two, put a baby in a stroller, etc. Now he's at it for a half-hour at a time. And he was completely nonverbal a year ago. We're just leaping through these developments.

He's sleeping at night, whether or not he naps. He's drinking lots and lots of juice and water, which is delightful. I've always worried that he was dehydrated because he drank so little and his urine always looked so dark. His aversions and sensory issues are greatly improved. All of a sudden he will eat the ends of bananas. He'll eat new things. He rejects them at first but after a few presentations, he tries them. He tolerates things he used to hate, like having to listen to me talking with teachers and ignoring him for an hour! My advice to anyone is to follow the diet fanatically and trust it. Let go of the other stuff. You can always go back if you find that there are bad results from quitting. I've always believed that my son could recover and would if we could find the right approach, and now I feel absolutely positive that we've found it.

Thanks from the bottom of my heart to everyone here, especially Elaine.

E. We have been on SCD (OK, a few goof ups!) since February. I knew if I asked my hubby to change our son's diet he would not want to. So I said, let's try it for 10 days and see if it makes a difference.

* * * *

Dr. Baker: *This is a really important point. Trying a diet for 10 days is definitely a good way to sell an idea that may otherwise be hard to swallow. The autism world that I know fosters a tendency to promote the most difficult ways of doing things just as it tolerates the magnification of small truths. It's as if the initiation of new parents to the biomedical club requires them to be frightened and intimidated by how hard it will be to do everything. In a way, that is understandable because generous intellectual, emotional, and financial resources are required by parents who follow this path as opposed to those who accept the "don't look for answers" path. Moreover, those of us who write books share Elaine Gottschall's inclination to set very strict standards for compliance to minimize the chance that readers will say, "Oh, I tried that and it didn't work," because they didn't do it right.*

It may take as long as a year to be sure that a gluten-free diet is not working. It may take as long as three months to know that a casein-free diet is not working. I have yet to figure out how long it takes to know that SCD is not working. But the fact is that changes that we make for our kids usually show their ultimate benefits in the first week or so—at least with sufficient clarity to encourage extending the trial.

Part of the gain from trying something new comes from the exercise of the courage and intention that change requires. The healing effects of courage and intention make for a lot of confusion. Patients often ask me, "If we are doing two or more things at once, how will we know what is working?" There are two answers to this very good question. One is that if the things we are doing are without risk of reactions that force a time-consuming retreat, then we are only chancing the confusion of success, which we can deal with later. Another answer is that every single thing we do is not single. Any new supplement, medication, diet, or therapy is joined by intention, which itself has its own healing power. That being said, we must remember that what is at stake is never the truth, or proof, or absolute confidence of permanent commitment. We just want to find a path to a higher elevation from which to view our landscape and perfect our navigation.

Choosing the biomedical path requires a commitment, but I think that many people have a problem with the commitment because they are overwhelmed by violating professional advice not to look for answers, and because they see the biomedical approach as one huge, confusing task—like cleaning up two generations worth of junk in your parents' attic. The best answer to such a task is to take it one small step at a time, letting the rewards of small advances boost the small intention embodied in the first step. Some parents, when told of the potential benefits of any treatment, are ready to move straight to warp speed. Many are intimidated by a big commitment that lacks the guarantees that appear to come from the small commitment of filling a prescription for a drug. It helps a lot to remember that the true obstacle is not the impossibility of changing what your kid eats, but overcoming your fear of failure. Try it for one day, two days, three days. Mother Nature is quite forgiving. If you drop the ball, you can pick it up and try again.

* * * *

We did it over winter break. Sam did not "recover" in 10 days. He is seven years old and high-functioning autistic (HFA). BUT... he was so much calmer, less irritable, and better at transitions better that after just 10 days my darling hubby said, "We can do this forever if it helps his attitude this much." We have seen many new skills emerge this year and I attribute most of them to SCD. My advice is to present the diet as a trial. My husband was sold in 10 days but if he hadn't been, I would have tried something like, "Let's just give it a month to make sure...." Also, plan menus, put all the non-SCD food in the garage (after all, it's only a trial, you can't throw it out yet!), and have everyone eat SCD at home. If they can't take it, let hubby take the others out for a sneaky treat of PIZZA. We eat basically SCD at home and when in Rome... HFA son eats SCD 100% (OK, there have been a few slip-ups). His eye contact is improved. He rides his bike more independently. He can now wear a bike helmet (sensory problem with this previously). He actually looks at other children now to see what they are doing, previously no interest. He can imitate in a sort of "follow me" game. *He sleeps by himself every night!* I thought I was going to have him in our bed until he was at least 10 and then Daddy was going to sleep with him. I have my bed back! I never thought that would happen. He transitions very well. Previously, he tantrummed at transitions whether it was an activity he enjoyed or not. He can tolerate the dog sitting with him. He would push her away before. I think this is another sensory issue. He can take "no" for an answer. He can tolerate one-on-one time with his teachers better. He is participating more at calendar and circle times. He is still improving and his improvements have all been gradual. I am thrilled with this diet.

F. Six months back, my son's kindergarten team, along with a child psychologist, declared to us that our son Nicholas could be autistic as he fits the characteristics. We had some meetings with them and finally, in September, had a team of doctors evaluated him. The initial diagnosis was Asperger's, which [was later changed] to dyslexia. We were amazed at [the second] diagnosis as they could not identify autistic behavior in him. The only reason they gave was that he is trilingual so he is not coping with the situations around him. So there was a clear change in diagnosis. We believe that SCD has brought a big change in his behavior. He is completely different than before, learning a lot. The most amazing thing is that he has started playing with other kids. I think all the credit goes to SCD.... I hope that with SCD he will continue improving. He has started differentiating between right and left, his backward alphabets are going forward now, and there are many other improvements. This is all because of SCD and goat milk yogurt.

G. Dear SCDers, In answer to the question re the four-year-old autistic child without stomach problems... I have had Asperger's syndrome since age one (from DPT shot). I am a grandparent now, so I don't need to tell you how old I am. Anyway, I never had stomach issues. However, I could not think straight, was always confused, did not comprehend spoken language well, was very clumsy, etc.... Of course, back in those days nobody knew about autism; you were just called stubborn and a pain in the neck (!!!). So I grew up (all messed up) and made more mistakes in life than you can shake a stick at.... And then I learned about autism and the SCD and other therapies. I started the SCD on July 31, 2003. By the sixth day my dizziness started to go away. By day eight, I was only dizzy in the morning and the confusion started to lift. By the tenth day, I was able to comprehend verbal language much better and to express myself verbally without having my thoughts fly out of my head in the middle of a sentence (which had been happening in nearly every conversation I had). So, in answer to the question about your four-year-old, in my opinion, even though there appear to be no stomach issues, the SCD will be a big help for recovery and development for your child. It's an easy diet, healthful and delicious, so why not give it a try... you may be pleasantly surprised by the results. It certainly won't hurt.

H. I just wanted to give a brief rundown of some of the major improvements Miguel has experienced during his seven and a half months on SCD.

NO meltdowns—they were pretty common before, even on GFCF. Now he has small short tantrums every once in a while that seem very age-appropriate. This improvement happened almost immediately. We can go anywhere now, even festivals and the mall!

Initiates play with other children and adults—this has been improving since day one, too. Has reached the level of initiating games of hide-and-go-seek and chase!

Much more spontaneous language—this one has been steadily improving and has now reached the stage of five-word sentences with correct use of pronouns! He also engages in conversational-type language and answers questions—appropriately!

Engages others in snuggling and hugging—this morning Miguel and I were still in bed (talking!) and DH came in to say goodbye. He bent down and Miguel put one arm around Tim's neck and one arm around mine and pulled our three heads together for a joint nuzzle. Bliss!

Greets people spontaneously—when my dad or grandmother used to enter a room, Miguel would truly ignore their greetings. He would just turn his head and literally pretend not to hear. Now, he greets them first, or in response—happily and enthusiastically. He always gives hugs good-bye and waves from the driveway. He even waved hello and called out, "Hi, Josh," the other day—across the school driveway to a *former* classmate.

Pretend play and no perseveration with non-toy items—he makes his trains and animals talk to each other with spontaneous dialogue (not scripting). He has his dinosaurs pretend to eat little balls he is calling dinosaur food—they came with a different toy for a different purpose. This kind of thing *never* happened pre-SCD and has steadily improved. He used to obsess on non-toy objects... not any more.

Well, that's a lot and not really all there is to tell. I haven't even touched on the physical differences. Maybe another time. Miguel was probably somewhere in the moderate range on the spectrum pre-SCD—verbal, but almost exclusively scripting. The only improvements on GFCF (six months prior) were better eye contact and a little less fog. He lived on waffles, cookies, and french fries, soy milk, and apple juice, and had horrific BMs. I honestly thought that was the healthy thing for him... I was so naive!!

I. I will tell you that the GAINS he has made, well it is so worth staying on this diet!!!!!! Let me repeat that: the GAINS he has made make it so worth staying on this diet!!!!!! He is much more verbal than ever before, his response time has markedly decreased, his eye contact and overall attention are *much* better. His tantrums are *gone* altogether.

Lest you think we have been at this long, I will tell you that we have only been completely SCD for *only* three weeks!

J. My little daughter Rachael, who is twenty and a half months old, has been having seizures since she turned eight and a half months—following her third set of immunizations.

We tried drugs—and they made things worse. Then we tried the SCD but never took dairy out, and her seizures got significantly better. But instead of continuing with the SCD, we decided to try the ketogenic diet next, which has been designed to control seizures. It too made things worse.

As we were coming off the ketogenic diet in October, I decided to switch Rachael to the SCD but this time to follow the ASD protocol, and substitute goat dairy for cow dairy. Her seizures, which she had had every day for 363 days, stopped five days after putting her on the cow-dairy-free SCD. I thought that those days would never come.

It has been about 12 days since her seizures stopped, and Rachael is developing again and doing things that she has never done—making more effort to communicate, playing with toys more appropriately. She is alert and occasionally more cranky—she makes her feelings known, which is a very good thing.

The change is amazing, her personality is coming back and we cannot contain our joy!!!! We pray that this is a permanent cessation of seizures and that as long as we keep on this diet, her brain will heal and she will make a complete recovery.

Thank you Elaine and everyone else who takes the time to share the information re this amazing diet.

K. I want to give everyone an update on my son, Zachary. A little background—he was diagnosed mild ASD or developmental delay with autistic traits a year ago. He has been GFCF for almost one year. He made dramatic improvements the first few months on GFCF but leveled off sometime after that. He has not had any major gastrointestinal issues but has had some problems with constipation. I don't have him on any supplements now except for calcium and magnesium and we haven't tried the yogurt yet.

The first few weeks we were on SCD, the only change I noticed was that his moods seemed more even and he seemed more calm. During the third week, I began to feel that he was consistently understanding me better and that his comments, although they were only short phrases, were all making sense! Prior to SCD, he would have days where he understood me and made sense followed by days where I felt I was talking to a brick wall and he just wasn't able to communicate.

Sometime during the fourth week, he began surprising me with new words and phrases. It is rare to hear him say anything new, let alone new words every day! His speech teacher recently tested him in an area that he had just been tested in six weeks ago. Six weeks ago, he scored poorly enough that there was a goal made on his IEP related to this test. When she retested him a week ago, he scored 19 out of 20. She made a comment about how great he is doing receptively. We have not told her about the diet.

During this last week, he was consistently using sentences with seven and eight words, and in the last few days he used complex sentences of 10 to 15 words. I have never heard him use sentences like this. Even when he is using shorter sentences, he will say a couple of them in a row to string his thoughts together. We are having simple conversations for the first time! Prior to SCD, he had been using a single five-to-six-word sentence or short phrase to communicate.

I am still having a hard time absorbing the fact that this diet is helping him tremendously. I think I am just afraid it will stop. How can something so simple have such a profound effect on my child and why were we so blessed to stumble upon it?

Thank you Elaine for your book!

L. There is a definite change in his behavior for the better! He is starting to communicate with us by trying to ask for something when he needs to and also by writing notes to us. His voice is starting to come out again, and even though it sounds croaky from lack of use, it is so wonderful to hear it! Before SCD, he had not talked or made one sound in over two months. He is also starting to be creative again, for example, making and labeling little boxes for us to put items in; also, he is starting to draw again like he used to. He is actually so aware of everything around him, listening to everything we say, and we can verify that because he will type into the computer the things we were talking about, and he can find them. He is also reading every magazine that is around him. He reads a lot!

He has actually been off all antihistamines for the entire month he has been on SCD, and it does not seem like he really needs them anymore. The chronic runny nose he had all these past seven years is nearly gone.

His color is so much better; it is as if he is getting more oxygen in his blood. He doesn't have that sallow, pasty color anymore, and he has more energy now. Even his fingers, which previously looked so skinny, look a little better, as if there is a little more fat on them.

Elaine, you have no idea how severely autistic my son was. He was completely normal at age 12; but went into a continuous regression after the

MMR vaccine booster at that age until he was completely inhibited into a frozen, stiff 19-year-old teenager who was losing weight. That is how he was right before starting SCD.

Of all the treatments we have done on him over the last seven years, my husband and I agree that this is the most improvement we have seen in him in such a short time (one month on SCD). He is actually starting to come out of his inhibited shell in so many ways. This is so amazing! Thanks so much Elaine for giving us this diet. You are giving my son his life back as well as ours.

M. All I can say is I am so very grateful. :) Thank you, Elaine.... Today I truly saw the baby boy who had slipped away from me. He is bright, alert, laughing, imitating speech, initiating funny play, and laughing at it himself... he is "there" again. It is funny how I did not see how he had slipped away so much... just because I in the middle of it, I'm sure.

We had made great strides on casein-free and started this diet only a week or so ago rather than starting gluten-free. He is eating foods I never thought he would eat and has almost overcome the sensory issues that were so serious. We are not nearly to the end of this but today I was able to truly enjoy his precious personality again... and so was he. What a gift to give back to a child and a family. Thank you again... I am sure that there will be many more hurdles and days that are not so good, but it has put this Mother on her knees today to see that this little boy is still "in there" and that hopefully we can continue to progress and regain lost ground.

Thanks again... hoping for good news and steady progress with all these deserving children and adults. And most of all I pray that parents who have not tried this will give their children the chance to improve by using the diet and toughing out the difficult moments. I know we have much yet ahead of us but hearing that laugh gives the incentive to keep pushing on.

Thank you Elaine... I know one little boy who can now have a normal life hopefully... and a mother, who waited 20 years on a child, who can see a way to have this precious child "back" again. There is no way to thank you or this group for the part you played in that.

CHAPTER VI

Today

To the greatest Dr. Mom of them all....

The top 10 reasons why we love Dr. Moms and the Specific Carbohydrate Diet:

10. You get to talk about your child's poops all day.
9. You get to talk about other kids' poops all day
8. You get to bake muffins at 11:00 at night when you suddenly realize that you don't have enough for the next day.
7. You get to meet a load of people just as insane as you, and talk about poop all day.
6. You get to spend $1,500 on groceries, $1,400 of that on almond flour.
5. You get to know the people in your health food store like family... and tell them all about your kid's poop.
4. You rapidly become a five-star chef.
3. You get to lord it over your friends who still feed their kids crap like McDonald's.
2. You get to talk about your child's poop all day.
1. You get to watch your child heal.

Thank you, Elaine.

With love,
Dr. Moms

– from a plaque we "Dr. Moms" made for Elaine, which I presented at her first DAN! conference

I told you at the start of this book that it really has no ending. Maybe, someday, I'll be able to write a sequel, which, as one of my friends suggested to me, will begin, "Alex, now a handsome and healthy 20-year-old..." But for now, I have to conclude with the truth of where we are today:

I recently sat on the couch working on my laptop. Alex was watching a video. (The fact that he now chooses to spend his time with us in the same room, rather than go off on his own to flap and squeak in the corner of the basement, is in itself pretty huge.) He came over to sit next to me, snuggled into my side, and the two of us sat there for well over an hour. We sat together, me and my son. Periodically, he'd lean his head into mine to cuddle and play with my hair a little... and I suddenly realized that we were at peace. Alex and I sat together at peace. No pain. No insanity. Peace.

For an hour of peace with my son, I have had to fight for every one of the 13 years of his life. I thought to myself, I will finish this book. I will do whatever it takes to make myself as knowledgeable as possible so I can help Alex and any other child who needs me. I will do my best to follow in Elaine's broad footsteps, even though I'm just me. Because the world really is better for her "glorious quest" and I'm nothing if not tenacious....

It is the mission of each true knight...
To dream the impossible dream,
To fight the unbeatable foe,
To bear with unbearable sorrow,
To run where the brave dare not go;
To right the unrightable wrong.
To love, pure and chaste, from afar,
To try, when your arms are too weary,
To reach the unreachable star!

This is my Quest to follow that star,
No matter how hopeless, no matter how far,
To fight for the right
Without question or pause,
To be willing to march into hell
For a heavenly cause!

– from *Man of LaMancha*

* * * *

Dr. Baker: *After I first understood its underlying science and saw the benefits of SCD in my patients and myself, I came to the belief that it was pretty much how I and everyone should eat all the time and for all time. Now, a few years later, I believe that SCD is a healing diet that should be let go once it—and other measures—have broken the vicious cycle that was its target. That was, after all, what Elaine Gottschall meant by the title of her book. I take refuge in this point in order to escape having to simultaneously reconcile all the diets that make up the menu of options for our children on the autism spectrum (and for individuals with other chronic illnesses in which the gut is the center of inflammation with systemic consequences).*

Gluten-free, casein-free, low-oxalate, salicylate- and phenolic-free, SCD, vegan diets are actually possible in families with an ethos that is intolerant of food refusal and in children with good appetites and relatively few sensory issues involving food tastes and textures. Another requirement is a parent who has the intellectual, emotional, and financial resources to do the homework, spend the time, and find support from other parents who have climbed this mountain. The emotional resources I refer to are not necessarily nice emotions. Start with guilt and add some fear and anger—some of which stem from outrages experienced in doctors' offices. The movement that Bernard Rimland began has gained momentum from the collective energy of pissed-off moms. Judy embodies all of those emotions and, with the help of her collaborating Dr. Mom parents, has generously and passionately and constructively shared them in this book to inform and inspire you—just as she has inspired me over the years of a relationship formed for the purpose of trying to do the best for Alex.

When I was just out of medical school, my first rotation in my pediatric internship at Yale was at the Southbury Training School, which housed hundreds of children and adults with serious developmental problems. In 1964, Southbury was widely admired as a model institution, and I was fortunate to have the example of Dr. Roy Breg, Dr. Herman Yannet, and others of its staff. A pediatric resident, Leandro Cordero, freshly arrived from Argentina, was my fellow medical house officer, as interns and residents are known. After evening rounds, in conversations that gave room for personal stories, philosophy, and reflection, Leo made a simple comment that startled me with its frank simplicity: "Medicine is a way of giving love." Not exactly Yale sort of talk! The talk stuck with me, and resonates when I think of the emotional resources that Judy has devoted to channeling the collective energy of the Dr. Moms. So, if someone asks you what Judy's book is all about, "love" would be a good answer.

My commentary is the result of Dr. Rimland's suggestion that I add my perspective to Judy's. With that in mind, let me close with this comment about a passion that Bernie and I shared: letting the data talk.

We live in a world in which the truth is thrown down upon us from above. "They" tell us what has been proven and unproved; what is trustworthy and what is doubtful. Our survival as individuals and professionals depends to a large extent on our presumption of the integrity and timeliness of those who feed the pipeline that delivers our personal and public truths. By "timeliness" I mean that information is contemporary with current experience, which may not be found in libraries where public policy is forged.

Dr. Rimland began in the 1960s to devise a technology for the contemporary medical experience of individuals and families to be given a voice—a means of collecting their wisdom about what is and is not working for them, so that others like them could obtain guidance. The key words here are "like them," which is an awkward concept, considering that each of us is unique. Nevertheless, Bernie's innovation of a system for tabulating and reporting responses to questions about "what has worked for your child?" has provided a rich resource for parents of children whose common ground was the imprecise label "autism." Stephen Edelson, Ph.D., Dr. Rimland's collaborator in the collection, tabulation, and reporting of parental responses, continues the project as he continues the leadership of the Autism Research Institute.

In the 1990s, Judy and I worked together to launch a project that offers an advanced Internet-based project with the same goals. This system, Medigenesis. com, is, as this book goes to press, re-emerging from an eclipse that began with the bursting of the dot-com bubble. Check with www.AutismWebsite.com for more details about a resource with the same intention as ARI and Judy's book: to bring to you the experience of other families confronting problems like yours.

The pipeline from which this experience of other families is distilled is not the high altitude of the government, academia, and the pharmaceutical industry but the contemporary collective experience conveyed to us by the data of people like us. The general picture that we have obtained from the parents, physicians, and researchers in the Defeat Autism Now! community tells us that autism is a digestive system problem in which the brain's difficulties in taking in and processing the environment are a downstream result of the same kinds of troubles in the gut. Autism: Effective Biomedical Treatments, by Jon Pangborn and me, presents that picture in more detail as we try to find better *ways of answering for each child the vexing question that Judy confronted as she followed a path that led to the Specific Carbohydrate Diet: "Have we done everything we can for this child?"*

That question is more daunting than the traditional question—"Have we done what 'they' say should be done for autism?"—because the strategy is based on different principles. Those principles are individuality, balance, and control. Recognizing the individuality of each person places an enormous burden on those charged with unraveling puzzles of that person's health. Protocols for managing a disease restrict treatment options based on the few ways individuals in a group are similar, and ignore the ways they differ. Individuality demands two questions based on the second principle: balance. Those two questions have to do with whether this individual has unmet special needs to get certain substances or to avoid, or be rid of certain allergens or toxins. Those questions demand the application of a third principle: control. By "control" I refer to the question of who decides. In complex chronic illness, should the clinician be the sole person to make all the decisions and the parents and child remain passively obedient to his or her choices? No. The more complex the terrain, the more collaborative must be the efforts to leave no stone unturned. The medical model for treating acute medical emergency may appropriately put the physician in full control. Chronic illness demands a collaborative effort in which the clinician is the guide and the parents and child are the scouts. In this model the patient is the real expert who reveals the best choices by his or her lab results and response to diagnostic trials. In this model the physician is the teacher, who in the end learns the most from the successes and failures encountered in a relationship with patients in which both are changed.

* * * *

Here I am now, writing the final chapter of the book Elaine and I envisioned two years ago. In January of 2006, I enrolled in a master's degree program in holistic nutrition. If Elaine could go back to get an undergraduate degree when she was 49 or so, I certainly can find a way to get another advanced degree at 42! My first goal to first get this book published, in the hope that the sooner it is, the sooner it will be available to help families. My second goal is to finish this degree as rapidly as possible, so I can better help children on the spectrum and their families. My third immediate goal is to do whatever I can to forward the cause of SCD by helping, whenever and wherever possible, to promote awareness of it.

And of course, while I do all this, I will try to make Alex get better still.

I like to set lofty goals for myself. It keeps me on my toes.

I have always tried to live by the mantra, "If it can't hurt and it could help, I will do it." Accordingly, I never stop looking for new things to try. Daily, I talk to moms to learn what they are learning, to see what they are reading, to hear what they are thinking.

SCD is not the whole answer. Of course, as with any treatment, there are always going to be those children who respond so dramatically so as to be cured by this approach alone. I do not doubt the stories parents tell about their children's near-miraculous recoveries from this diet. I have seen it myself. But I have been around the block too many times to think that there is one answer to the autism puzzle. Alex was diagnosed more than 11 years ago. This past decade saw me try hundreds of treatments, almost all of which failed. I am still out there, knee-deep in mud in the trenches, looking for answers and fighting the enemy.

But SCD worked. SCD got my son out of his agony. SCD has given his life joy, and in the process, given my life meaning. While I hate fanaticism of any kind, I will admit to being somewhat fanatical about SCD. Having now seen child after child feel better and better and better, it is both a forgivable and understandable fault in me.

The way I look at things, we always have a choice. For example, sure, I could stop fighting for Alex and have a lot more time (and money) for myself. But if I do that then I am accepting that this is the rest of his life. No, I don't accept that. I believe that he has great intelligence and that if I can rid his body of its poisons, whatever they may be, I will in turn be giving his brain a chance to heal as well. I will be giving that intelligent, sensitive, loving, and lovely human being a chance to become what he should have been.

That leads me to mention one more thought I often have. Whenever I feel like I can't go on one more day, I pull myself out of my "black pit of despair" by focusing on the good that has come into my life from autism. From even the worst things in the world, good can come. Because of autism, I have met some of the greatest human beings to have walked this earth. I had Elaine. I have been hugged by Bernard Rimland. I have the Dr. Moms, who are truly the most remarkable people I could ever imagine befriending. Most of all, perhaps, I think of friends who were helped by hearing about Alex's response to SCD. For example, I think of Sharie and Eric. What would have happened to Eric if I *hadn't* met them that day in the lab? When I think about Eric, my heart always gives an extra thump and my eyes water automatically. Did Alex and my presence there in the lab that day really help him to suffer less? And Candace and Zachary. Did that phone call really help get Zachary out of his agony? If even one of you reading this book decides to put your child on SCD, and your child stops screaming in pain, then yes, good and meaning have come from Alex's suffering.

And I know that he would want that to be the case.

For all of you out there who still have doubts, I will end with a little story sent to me recently by my friend Heather, whose son's life was undoubtedly saved by SCD (read their story in Chapter 5). I have said over and over that SCD is not easy. It means an effort on your part to help your child. The truth is that in the end, as they begin to get well, your children will know and understand.

> *Judy, I know that Aidan still has so much more healing to do. But he still loves me. My boy, who had turtle meatballs with cold beets for breakfast on the way to school, still loves me. In spite of everything I have had to do to him. When it was time to give one of the hundred remedies he gets a day, he said to me, "Mommy, thank you for healing me."*

Footnotes

[1] Kingsley, E P. *Welcome to Holland.* c1987.

[2] Wakefield, A J; Murch, S H; Anthony, A; Linnell, J; Casson, D M; Malik, M; Berelowitz, M; Dhillon, A P; Thomson, M A; Harcey, P; Valentine, A; Davies, S E; Walker-Smith, J A. Ileal-lymphoid-nodular hyperplasia, non-specific colitis, and pervasive developmental disorder in children. *Lancet* 1998; 351 (9103): 637-641.

[3] Uhlmann, V; Martin, C M; Sheils, O; Pilkington, L; Silva, I; Killalea, A; Murch, S B; Walker-Smith, J; Thomson, M; Wakefield, A J; O'Leary, J J. Potential viral pathogenic mechanism for new variant inflammatory bowel disease. *Molecular Pathology* 2002 April; 55(2): 84-90.

[4] Pangborn, J; Baker, S M. *Autism: Effective Biomedical Treatments.* 2005.

[5] Hall, R. *Psychiatric Adverse Drug Reactions: Steroid Psychosis.* Dr. Richard C.W. Hall Publications.

[6] Translation from the Greek by Ludwig Edelstein. From *The Hippocratic Oath: Text, Translation, and Interpretation,* by Ludwig Edelstein. Baltimore: Johns Hopkins Press, 1943.

[7] http://www.geocities.com/everwild7/noharm.html

[8] http://www.aamc.org

[9] Pangborn, J; Baker, S M. *Autism: Effective Biomedical Treatments.* 2005.

[10] Pangborn, J; Baker, S M. *Autism: Effective Biomedical Treatments.* 2005., p. 36-37.

[11] http://www.gao.gov/cghome/hccrisis/img40.html

[12] http://www.cnn.com/HEALTH/9907/15/kid.vaccine/

[13] http://www.cdc.gov/nip/publications/fs/rotavirus.htm

[14] http://www.health-care-reform.net/causedeath.htm

[15] http://www.cdc.gov/nip/vacsafe/concerns/cancer/default.htm

[16] *The New York Times*, December 1, 1964.

[17] *The New York Times*, February 14, 1960.

[18] Prasad, R. (2002). *Colitis and Me: A Story of Recovery.* New Haven: SCD Recipe LLC.

[19] Institute for Functional Medicine, 13th annual symposium, Tampa, FL